The Young Adult Chronic Patient

Bert Pepper, Hilary Ryglewicz, *Editors*

NEW DIRECTIONS FOR MENTAL HEALTH SERVICES
H. RICHARD LAMB, *Editor-in-Chief*

Number 14, June 1982

Paperback sourcebooks in
The Jossey-Bass Social and Behavioral Sciences Series

Jossey-Bass Inc., Publishers
San Francisco • Washington • London

The Young Adult Chronic Patient
Number 14, June 1982
     Bert Pepper, Hilary Ryglewicz, *Editors*

New Directions for Mental Health Services Series
H. Richard Lamb, *Editor-in-Chief*

New Directions for Mental Health Services (publication number
USPS 493-910) is published quarterly by Jossey-Bass Inc.,
Publishers. Second-class postage rates paid at San Francisco,
California, and at additional mailing offices.

Correspondence:
Subscriptions, single-issue orders, change of address notices,
undelivered copies, and other correspondence should be sent to
New Directions Subscriptions, Jossey-Bass Inc., Publishers,
433 California Street, San Francisco, California 94104.

Editorial correspondence should be sent to the Editor-in-Chief,
H. Richard Lamb, Department of Psychiatry and the Behavioral
Sciences, U.S.C. School of Medicine, 1934 Hospital Place,
Los Angeles, California 90033.

Library of Congress Catalogue Card Number LC 81-48483
International Standard Serial Number ISSN 0193-9416
International Standard Book Number ISBN 87589-908-0

Cover art by Willi Baum
Manufactured in the United States of America

Ordering Information

The paperback sourcebooks listed below are published quarterly and can be ordered either by subscription or as single copies.

Subscriptions cost $35.00 per year for institutions, agencies, and libraries. Individuals can subscribe at the special rate of $21.00 per year *if payment is by personal check.* (Note that the full rate of $35.00 applies if payment is by institutional check, even if the subscription is designated for an individual.) Standing orders are accepted.

Single copies are available at $7.95 when payment accompanies order, and *all single-copy orders under $25.00 must include payment.* (California, Washington, D.C., New Jersey, and New York residents please include appropriate sales tax.) For billed orders, cost per copy is $7.95 plus postage and handling. (Prices subject to change without notice.)

To ensure correct and prompt delivery, all orders must give either the *name of an individual* or an *official purchase order number.* Please submit your order as follows:

Subscriptions: specify series and subscription year.
Single Copies: specify sourcebook code and issue number (such as, MHS8).

Mail orders for United States and Possessions, Latin America, Canada, Japan, Australia, and New Zealand to:
Jossey-Bass Inc., Publishers
433 California Street
San Francisco, California 94104

Mail orders for all other parts of the world to:
Jossey-Bass Limited
28 Banner Street
London EC1Y 8QE

New Directions for Mental Health Services Series
H. Richard Lamb, *Editor-in-Chief*

MHS1 *Alternatives to Acute Hospitalization,* H. Richard Lamb
MHS2 *Community Support Systems for the Long-Term Patient,* Leonard I. Stein
MHS3 *Mental Health Consultations in Community Settings,* Alexander S. Rogawski
MHS4 *Coping with the Legal Onslaught,* Seymour Halleck
MHS5 *Adolescence: Perspectives on Psychotherapy,* Sherman Feinstein
MHS6 *Crisis Intervention in the 1980s,* Gerald F. Jacobson
MHS7 *The Fairweather Lodge: A Twenty-Five Year Retrospective,*
George W. Fairweather
MHS8 *Middle Management in Mental Health,* Stephen L. White
MHS9 *Perspectives on Rural Mental Health,* Morton O. Wagenfeld

Contents

Editors' Notes

The imperfect label "young adult chronic patient," originally the title of a conference in Rockland County, New York, in 1980, has come into common use in our professional vocabulary. It attempts to describe a generation of young adults in the age group eighteen to thirty-five who show persistent and severe impairment in their psychological and social functioning. They are our first generation of severely disabled psychiatric patients to grow up in the community, under policies which we have called the flip side of deinstitutionalization: policies of admissions diversion and short-stay hospitalization which are directed toward protecting potential patients' civil rights and allowing them to live in the least restrictive environment.

Unfortunately, that environment — the community — is not only least restrictive but often least supportive. If and when they are hospitalized, their stays are brief, and typically they are discharged when their most acute symptoms have subsided, but they are still in a vulnerable state of incomplete remission. They are discharged back into lives which do not support their recovery: into families wracked by tension and conflict but serving as their principal or only resource; into board-and-care homes occupied by older, chronic, deinstitutionalized patients and the elderly; or into the cheerless rooms of welfare hotels, where they try to live without jobs, without friends, and, commonly, without hope.

These patients are ill-equipped to make use of existing treatment and support services; they are often insufficiently monitored or, in effect, rejected by service systems. They are often too withdrawn or disruptive to be readily engaged in treatment. They make inappropriate use — underuse, overuse, misuse, abuse — of treatment programs and clinicians; or, to view it another way, our services are not designed to fill their needs.

In November, 1980, the Rockland County Community Mental Health Center (CMHC) and the Albany Institute for Education and Training co-sponsored a ground-breaking conference on the Young Adult Chronic Patient in Suffern, New York, which was attended by more than 400 mental health professionals. This conference was repeated in an expanded form in Albany, in June 1981. The chapters in this volume, with two exceptions (Chapters Three and Four) are based on presentations made at those two conferences. The first four chapters are directed primarily at defining the population and presenting research results and accounts of clinical experience at four locations in New York State. The next seven chapters (including five brief accounts of treatment programs at the Rockland County Community Mental Health Center) are essentially discussions of treatment. The volume concludes with a discussion of model programs and their applicability to this patient group, and

1

a philosopher's perspective on issues in mental health service delivery. Two of the chapters (Sheets, Prevost, and Reihman; Bachrach) have been published in *Hospital and Community Psychiatry* (March, 1982), and some of the research material in the first chapter (Pepper and Ryglewicz) was published in a special section of the July, 1981, issue of *Hospital and Community Psychiatry* devoted to the young adult chronic patient in the community (Pepper, Kirshner, and Ryglewicz, 1981).

The two conferences at which most of these papers were presented have marked the beginning of a lively and ongoing discussion, in conference presentations and in print, on the subject of this difficult patient group. This volume should be regarded as an attempt to document the opening statements of that conversation, which has already gone beyond these limits. We regret that space does not permit us to include still other perspectives on this problem, from other parts of the country and from other viewpoints, such as those emphasizing alternative and less traditional forms of care. It is our hope that these perspectives will be the subject of a future issue.

Bert Pepper
Hilary Ryglewicz
Editors

Reference

Pepper, B., Kirshner, M., and Ryglewicz, H. "The Young Adult Chronic Patient: Overview of a Population." *Hospital and Community Psychiatry*, 1981, *32*, 463–469.

Bert Pepper is a psychiatrist, director of the Rockland County Community Mental Health Center (Pomona, New York), clinical professor of psychiatry at New York University, and chairman of the New York State Conference of Local Mental Hygiene Directors.

Hilary Ryglewicz, ACSW, is clinical assistant to the director at the Rockland County Community Mental Health Center.

*Our first generation of young adult chronic psychiatric patients
since deinstitutionalization has emerged in the community.
Updated research results and case studies show different patterns
of emergence but similar indications for clinician response.*

The Uninstitutionalized Generation: A New Breed of Psychiatric Patient

Bert Pepper
Hilary Ryglewicz
Michael C. Kirshner

Who is the young adult chronic patient? This unsatisfactory phrase, which has
spread from Rockland County into the professional language, is used to describe
a generation of young adults in the age group eighteen to thirty-five who are
now living in our communities, but who show persistent and severe impairment in their psychological and social functioning. They are young persons
who, as they grow older, require services from mental health and other social
agencies in a variety of ways and over a period of years. We have called them
an emerging, uninstitutionalized generation; many of them are persons who
in the past would have become long-stay patients in mental institutions, or at
the least would have had one or several hospitalizations of one or more years'
duration. Today, however, they spend little if any time in our psychiatric
institutions. The seriously emotionally disturbed person who has become ill in
the past fifteen or twenty years usually can measure his or her total length of
stay in state institutions and other hospitals in weeks or months rather than in
years and decades. Even the schizophrenic patient who has been hospitalized
three times in the past ten years probably has spent perhaps 12 months in hospitals, and 108 months in the community. These young adults, then, are our

B. Pepper, H. Ryglewicz (Eds.). *New Directions for Mental Health Services: The Young Adult
Chronic Patient*, no. 14. San Francisco: Jossey-Bass, June 1982.

first generation of chronic psychiatric patients to grow up in community care and in the wake of the great wave of deinstitutionalization and its corollaries: admissions diversion, tightened involuntary admission criteria, and the limitation of hospital stays to the briefest possible time.

Many of these patients are diagnosed schizophrenic, and many others carry a diagnosis of other major mental or personality disorder. Many are multiply diagnosed — especially since the advent of DSM-III (Diagnostic and Statistical Manual of Mental Disorders [Third Edition], 1980) — with symptoms of mental illness superimposed on an underlying personality disorder. But our view of this patient group cuts across diagnostic lines, for our focus is on the functional disabilities of these young persons.

We may note here that the term *disability* itself refers to functioning, in this case functioning in the social context of a community (Gruenberg, 1982). The pathology of intrapsychic functioning, which constitutes an impairment which we may call mental illness or personality disorder, may not result in a disability in terms of living in a mental institution or being cared for as a dependent child in the context of one's family. But these impairments do constitute disabilities when the young adult attempts to become independent and self-supporting, to leave the protection of the family, to make stable relationships, and to live normally as a member of the community.

The constellation of symptoms that Gruenberg described two decades ago as social breakdown syndrome (poor social and psychological functioning, apathy, negativism, and docility mingled with episodic outbursts) was once seen, in part, as the product of the patient's interaction with the institutional environment — which was dull, understimulating, limited, predictable, protective, directive, and authoritarian (Gruenberg, 1963, 1966; Goffman, 1962). Today we see cases of social breakdown syndrome in the community context (Gruenberg and others, 1972; Gruenberg, 1974) — an environment that, by contrast, is exciting, overstimulating, open, unpredictable, dangerous, confusing, and demanding of choices by patients. The intrapsychic pathology of our young adult patients has not changed, but its expression has changed through their interaction with the community. Our problems with patients and responsibilities for their care are now different as well.

As caregivers, we find in young adult chronic patients the bane and despair of our working lives. Typically, they make poor use — underuse, overuse, misuse, abuse — of the services that are available. As perhaps 10 percent of our patient population, they consume perhaps 40 percent of our staff time. They tend not to define themselves as mental patients and do not have, unlike their older, long-institutionalized counterparts, years of training in doing as they are told (Segal, Baumohl, and Johnson, 1977; Segal and Baumohl, 1980). Instead, they want to be treated — and to act out — in the manner of their peers. They leave us as they leave their parents: with optimism or defiance, only to return again in crisis. They are typically our emergencies, our unexplained terminations, our no-shows, our unscheduled sessions, and our

AMA (Against-Medical-Advice) discharges. In a system such as Rockland County's, their charts are thick and have many sections, notes from several programs and clinicians, many beginnings and premature endings, and often two or three scribbled suicide notes. They are frustrating, difficult to treat, and often too withdrawn or disruptive to be readily engaged in treatment.

It may be too pessimistic to refer to all of these young persons as chronically disabled, although the phrase is accurate for many in the context of our present resources for treatment and support. These are the patients we may think of as our failures; certainly, failure is the most common element in their experience. They begin jobs, only to lose them; they begin school, only to drop out; they begin relationships, only to suffer additional conflict, dependency, and disappointment. Many try in vain to separate from their parents, but continually fall back into their reluctant embrace, seeking shelter, support, sustenance; many virtually withdraw from efforts to make it in the world; and many are engaged with their families in a repetitive cycle of hope, fear, rage, shame, and the recurrent violent conflict of prisoners locked together in a room with no exit.

If we look at these dysfunctional young adults in developmental terms, they seem to be stuck in the transition to adult life, unable to master the tasks of separation and independence. If we examine the nature of their failures, we find them to be based on more or less severe and chronic pathology: thought disorder; affective disorder; personality disorder; and severe deficits in ego functions such as impulse control, reality testing, judgment, modulation of affect, memory, mastery and competence, and integration. In terms of the necessary equipment for community life — the capacity to endure stress, to work consistently toward realistic goals, to relate to other people comfortably over time, to tolerate uncertainty and conflict — these young adults are disabled in a very real and pervasive sense.

Case Histories

Let us briefly introduce to your imagination three such young adults. These are all real persons, and their cases are not unusual.

(1) Sam is an attractive, curly-haired young man of twenty-seven whose poor self-image shows in his posture and his expression: His head is slightly lowered, his body poised as if for "fight or flight," and his look is mistrustful, a blend of sullenness and anxiety. Sam's problems did not emerge until late in high school, when he began using drugs and showed some personality change, becoming "belligerent and uncooperative." He first came to our crisis service at the age of eighteen, complaining, "I think I'm a moron." He had already attempted suicide more than once, usually under the influence of alcohol. He had a girlfriend, but felt unable to relate to her. He was still living at home with his parents — described as chronically in conflict, with Sam caught in the middle. He already had a history of drug abuse, smoking marijuana at times and experiencing paranoid episodes when

he took LSD. He was disorganized, preoccupied with daydreams, and concerned that he might be homosexual.

In the nine years following this episode, Sam has had seven psychiatric hospitalizations for anxiety, depression, confusion, and paranoid delusions; he has had multiple contacts with our crisis service and several referrals to our outpatient clinics. He has been treated at our acute day treatment program, referred to a vocational rehabilitation workshop, and placed at a residential farm for psychiatric patients, which he had to leave because of drinking. He has gone away to college but dropped out to return home; he has begun jobs but lost them because he would lie in bed in the morning. He has repeatedly been diagnosed schizophrenic and put on medication, but has repeatedly stopped his medications and dropped out of treatment. He has repeatedly returned to use of alcohol and marijuana, usually in connection with his efforts to make friends.

(2) Nick is a tall, thin, shy twenty-one-year-old who says he feels "like a jerk." He was born with a blood disease which necessitated a complete transfusion at birth. His family background includes an older brother who was hospitalized for psychiatric illness at an early age. Nick was in special classes from first grade until high school graduation, showing a dull-normal full-scale IQ with mild visual-motor problems, and severe, chronic feelings of inferiority. Since his parents' marital conflict culminated in divorce, he has been living with his father, who also appears depressed and withdrawn. Nick is diagnosed as mixed personality disorder with schizoid, paranoid, and avoidant features. He has been attending social and vocational rehabilitation programs since high school but still has great difficulty making social relationships. He was hospitalized recently when he became depressed about his future and tried to cut his wrists with the wires of his orthodontic braces.

(3) Nancy is a bright, bouncy, outspoken young woman of twenty-four who was able to complete two years of college and has had a few periods of successful work history as a therapy aide. She is cheerful, affectionate, likeable, full of fun, and full of life. She is also, at times, volatile, impatient, disruptive, profane, threatening, grandiose, and impulsive. She has had four psychiatric hospitalizations and is on lithium for manic-depressive illness, with an additional diagnosis of passive-aggressive personality. Nancy has abused drugs since age thirteen, starting with marijuana, glue-sniffing, cocaine and amphetamines, and more recently including alcohol. . . . Her problems in maintaining steady employment have resulted in severe financial crises, and her manic episodes have involved disastrous conflicts with landlords. Yet her intelligence and some successful work history make it very difficult for her to accept any lowering of her standard of living or of her hopes about the future. At present she is living in a transitional apartment and struggling to overcome her habitual use of drugs, which seems to play a part in precipitating her manic episodes.

These three young adults provide an idea of the range and variety of symptoms presented by our patient group, yet their social and treatment needs are in many ways strikingly similar. The most crippling aspects of their mental disorders are the effects of those disorders on the social functioning of these young persons and on their use, nonuse, or misuse of opportunities for treatment. When we strip away the pressure-sensitive diagnostic labels, their essential problem is that they cannot seem to get or keep anything positive going in their lives, including therapy.

In view of this, at the Rockland County Community Mental Health Center (CMHC) we have been pursuing a course of investigation designed to provide more data about young adult patients who show persistent difficulties in psychological and social functioning. We are also trying to develop a more precise understanding of the various routes by which these patients come to our attention, and the ages and stages at which they develop dysfunctional behavior.

The Center is the core agency of a unified services network which embraces the total care and treatment system for mentally ill, mentally retarded, developmentally disabled, alcoholic, and drug-abusing residents of our county of 270,000 persons. This large organization offers a natural habitat for studying young adults who are chronically mentally ill or socially disabled and for observing them in a variety of treatment programs.

We began with a very modest initial study of a segment of our own treatment population. From a group of 900 young adults in the age group eighteen to thirty who were seen at any of our six outpatient clinics within a three-month period in 1980, we identified, through input from clinicians and chart review, a group of nearly 300 who could be categorized as young adult chronic patients. This categorization was based on the severe and persistent nature of their disabilities and their dysfunctional use of treatment. Of these nearly 300 persons:

- 55 percent were male and 45 percent were female;
- 55 percent had mental health treatment before age eighteen;
- 25 percent had never been hospitalized;
- 60 percent were unemployed;
- 30 percent were receiving federal social security income based on disability;
- 27 percent were on public assistance;
- 19 percent were receiving support from their families; and only
- 24 percent were self-supporting;
- 24 percent were known to have been in trouble with the law;
- 37 percent had a known history of alcohol abuse, and 37 percent (not necessarily the same 37 percent) had a known history of marijuana abuse;
- 28 percent had a known history of other drug abuse; and for
- 42 percent of these persons, suicide had been an issue addressed in treatment.

We are now engaged in a more extensive effort to explore the size, nature, and needs of Rockland County's young adult chronic patient population. Of 1,200 young adults who had at least one contact with our Center in 1980 and at least one contact two years or more before, 800 were seen by their most recent clinicians as having the characteristics which define this patient group. We are now in the process of evaluating results of a questionnaire filled out by the clinicians of a sample of 250 of these 800 young adult chronic patients and those of a control group of nonchronic young adults. While the data must be verified through further analysis, preliminary results from a sub-sample of 100 of the chronic group suggests that:

- 69 percent had mental health treatment before age eighteen (47 percent outpatient, 22 percent inpatient);
- 55 percent are known by their clinicians to have used or abused one or a combination of alcohol and/or other drugs;
- 10 percent are known to have been involved in a criminal offense with violence;
- 5 percent are known to have been involved in a criminal offense without violence;
- 45 percent are still living with their families;
- 22 percent have their own children living with them, ranging in age from two to seventeen (for this group of 100 young adult patients, there were 44 such children living with their (22) parents;
- 31 percent are supported totally by some form of public assistance (including SSI — Supplementary Security Income);
- 8 percent receive public assistance supplementing part-time employment;
- 32 percent are supported by parents and/or spouse;
- 22 percent are self-supporting;
- 35 percent have made suicide attempts.

As noted elsewhere in this journal, the high suicide rate characteristic of this patient group becomes even more alarming when a city population is considered (Caton, 1981).

Based on both this developing exploratory study and our clinical observations of the young adult chronically disabled population, we would like to focus attention on two aspects of this patient group: first, the process of development of their problems; and, second, the process of their identification and treatment.

Evolution of the Problems

Our studies suggest that a majority of the young adult chronic patient population had received treatment before age eighteen. For some, like Nick, this means that problems were evident in childhood, and that some form of intervention was made even within the elementary school years. For others, the breakdown in functioning began in the adolescent years, sometimes in conjunction with the use of marijuana, alcohol, or other drugs as a part of recreational activity with peers. Our studies indicate that a majority of these young adults have a history of alcohol and marijuana abuse. There is some evidence accumulating that even brief use of marijuana may be a precipitating factor in psychotic episodes of persons who may be predisposed to develop a psychiatric disorder.

Certainly, it is observable in our own inpatient population that rehospitalizations often occur following ingestion of drugs. This becomes a thorny issue in treatment for our young adult chronic patients, who prefer to see their symptoms as a temporary reaction to drug use, and may say, "I used some bad stuff" or "Somebody slipped something into my drink," and yet strongly resist any implication that the recreational use of drugs enjoyed by their peers is off limits for them. Not only do they resist the idea that they are different and must observe a restriction because of a chronic vulnerability to certain kinds of stimuli, but many also find, in their use of drugs, their only respite from the demands of reality, and their only means of enjoying a commonality or making an effort to socialize with others of their age.

We do not know at this point what chemical interactions may be involved in the vulnerability to marijuana of young persons who have an underlying disorder which emerges in psychosis. But, considering the issue only in terms of ego functions, we can certainly surmise that drug use becomes abuse for young persons who have not been able to achieve other kinds of gratifications, and that a vicious cycle then ensues. The repeated retreat into drugs prevents the development of other satisfactions through goal-directed activity, and also prevents the working out of other issues such as the capacity to handle feelings of frustration, low self-esteem, and interpersonal conflict.

There is another and, again, very large group of young adult chronic patients whose breakdown in functioning appears only as the individual comes of age and attempts to separate from parents and to achieve autonomy. As we have noted before, the patient is stuck in the process of transition to adulthood. For some, functioning has been at least adequate through the high school years, but a breakdown has followed the attempt to go away to college, to marry, or to live with a girlfriend or boyfriend and, in particular, to become self-supporting—that is, to hold a job through consistent work activity. At this point, for many young persons, the personality structure proves inadequate to the new tasks of maturation into responsible adulthood. We know that young adulthood is often the time of the "first break" in schizophrenia. We are now seeing an apparent increase in the diagnosis of manic-depressive illness (bipolar disorder) in young persons, rather than the more typical picture of a manic disorder emerging in midlife. Again, we cannot say to what extent this seeming increase reflects an increased sensitivity to symptoms of mood disorder on the part of diagnosticians (following upon the availability and popularity of lithium), or an actual increase in emergence of the disorder at this earlier stage of life. The case of Nancy, whose use of drugs has become an increasingly obvious precipitant to her manic episodes, suggests a need for further research into the ramifications of the use of street drugs in the presence of a chronic chemical imbalance.

In the case of Sam (who apparently functioned well through high school, but showed a personality change at the time he became involved with drugs), we also do not know whether the functional change and the drug use were two reflections of the same difficulty—a breakdown in ego functions when confronting the tasks of separation and autonomy. It may be that the personality change and the development of severe anxiety and self-doubt were in fact secondary to the effects of drug use on a vulnerable individual with an underlying psychiatric disorder. As Sam has continued his course of multiple hospitalizations, his use of drugs and alcohol has presented an important element in the sabotage of efforts at rehabilitation—in one instance resulting in his discharge from a rehabilitative community.

The only other rural rehabilitative residences available for Sam would be those which focus on drug rehabilitation, which would not only be inappropriate for his needs but would demand a level of ego strength which he does not possess. Therefore, he falls between two chairs, as do many of the young adults whose dual (psychiatric and substance-abuse) diagnoses make them unwelcome referrals to many programs and also deserving of the term *multiply handicapped.*

Interactions with Treatment Programs

Having made these anecdotal observations of some of our young adult chronic patients, with clinical impressions of their process of entry into patienthood, what about the process of their interaction with treatment programs? Here, too, if we take not only a still shot but a movie, we see an initial episode of symptom development, whether in childhood or adolescence or young adulthood, which has an impact on family interactions and commonly results in treatment, either in the form of hospitalization or through outpatient programs. This first intervention, usually in a crisis, occurs in a context of maximum motivation and maximum optimism. Certainly, the episode comes as a shock to the young person and his significant others. But one episode is very different from six; the assumption, often encouraged by ourselves as professionals, is that functioning will be restored and even improved, and we often emphasize the advantage of this early warning signal, a sign that changes are needed in the life style and family interactions of the young person—and, of course, that therapy is indicated. The patient, too, tends to take an optimistic view at this early stage; unfortunately, much of the optimism is founded on denial. It is difficult to say, "This is what happened to me"; it feels better to say, "But it will never happen again." Often, the wish to forget it ever happened leads to a failure to follow through on therapy once the crisis or hospitalization is over. This may be as true of the family as of the patient. (Sam's mother, for instance, remains convinced that all of his troubles resulted from medicine he was given at our hospital.)

But by the second or third episode, especially if hospitalization is involved, it becomes more and more difficult to take an optimistic view of the future, both for the patient and for family and staff involved in his or her care. At this point, a growing pessimism among staff and family, as well as anger and resentment on some level, and a growing despair on the part of the patient become strong negative forces in the treatment picture. We might call this a rejection phase: The family and treatment staff reject the patient; the patient rejects himself as well as those who try to help him. Occasionally, we have the ultimate self-rejection, suicide, sometimes as the culmination of a postpsychotic depression, and sometimes resulting from an existential crisis and confrontation with a future devoid of hope.

Our therapeutic task as this process unfolds is to encourage enough recognition of the seriousness of the socially disabling disorder to motivate the patient and his family to follow through with treatment, and, at the same time, to mitigate the despair that sometimes accompanies this recognition. We want the patient and those around him to feel, on the one hand, that this is a very serious problem that needs attention but, on the other, that there is still hope. Achieving this balance is a delicate task of therapy. Helping patients and their families, as well as clinicians, to have appropriate expectations — not too much and not too little — is a still more delicate and equally necessary task. A striking feature of our young adult chronically disabled patients in the community is the discrepancy between the fantasy of what they would like to be able to do and the reality of what they have done and are likely to do in the future; it is the gap between the ideal of being "just like anybody else" and the reality of being unable to make anything work for very long.

Realistic Goals and Expectations

What goals can we realistically have for these dysfunctional young adults, which we can help them to identify and to share with us as therapists? And, once (hopefully) agreeing on appropriate goals, how can we tailor our treatment programs to move toward their realization?

Based on our observations of these patients, we can say that the following may be appropriate goals, both for individual clinicians and as the thrust or message of our treatment programs.

First, we must help them to become more self-aware and able to identify their own early warning signals of stress and impending chaos. Working toward this kind of self-awareness is not a matter of insight therapy; it is a sensitization to one's own signals. These signals may be behaviors, affective states, or cognitive patterns. For one individual, self-awareness may mean learning to say, "When I begin to have difficulty sleeping at night, it means that something is wrong." For another, it may mean, "When I start wanting to take on the whole world at once or thinking about becoming a rock star, I'm getting out of reality"; for another, "When I begin smoking a joint, when I feel anxious, I'm headed for trouble."

The second step in this kind of self-awareness is to identify something to do about these signals of overstress or impending decompensation. Calling one's therapist is one obvious response. Staying away from people who create stress or who present the temptation to fall back into drug and alcohol abuse is another. Moving to a less upsetting environment temporarily, but not running away completely, is another. Focusing on the performance of certain daily tasks, practicing relaxation or meditation techniques, or seeking out a trusted friend or relative are yet other ways of responding. The goal is to learn ways of achieving some degree of control over the kinds of stress and the kinds of temptation that have led in the past to a breakdown of functioning and a sense of helplessness.

A third aspect of self-awareness is the focusing of attention on certain core or repetitive problems, patterns of behavior that are dysfunctional and repeatedly lead the person into trouble. Examples are brooding about real or imaginary slights, procrastinating, or deciding after two weeks on a job that it is not the right job instead of sticking with it for the sake of sticking with something and overcoming the constant temptation to give up and run away.

Clearly, we are talking here about rather basic ego functions and elementary forms of everyday behavior. For many of these young adults, the therapist and the therapeutic group have to function as a borrowed ego to help with the functions of judgment, reality testing, memory, mastery and competence, and integration. This need is really at the core of our treatment of the young adult chronic patient. These young persons are like an organism which lacks the resources of the healthy human body. They are intensely vulnerable to the stresses of daily life because they do not have the ego strength to mobilize resistance to stress, to remember and integrate life experience, and to hold on to goals and intentions that are reality-based. The difficulty in mobilizing resources is not only psychological; it also interferes with patients' development of a social support network and with the constructive and appropriate use of treatment. Our first task, then, is to help them to develop their own ability and willingness to utilize help and support that is available. In the absence of both inner resources and the ability and willingness to utilize social supports, these young persons can only retreat under stress into patterns of withdrawal, drug abuse, fear, and rage.

A fourth and related aspect of self-awareness that these young persons need to develop is the focusing on realistic short-term expectations and goals. These patients need what we, as their clinicians, need: to be able to take satisfaction in limited, step-by-step achievements; to be able to say, "I've held on to this job for three weeks, and next week it will be four weeks," instead of "This job isn't getting me anywhere, and what I want to do is get a Ph.D. in psychology and help people." The other side of the coin of unrealistic and grandiose goals is, of course, the recognition of the goal as impossibly remote, and the despair of seeing reality as empty of hope and possibility. The one-day-at-a-time philosophy that has been so helpful in the treatment of alcohol addiction must become the focus of work with patients who are chronically tempted to run out on reality—if not into drugs, then into some other form of escape.

The issues noted above are examples, on the level of everyday life and everyday clinical management, of the ones we need to address with these persistently disabled young persons. What stands out as we try to address them in our treatment programs is that the same difficulties in continuity that these young persons show in their social functioning are an aspect, and often a fatal stumbling block, in their behavior as clients and their response to treatment. It is nearly impossible to help them to develop self-awareness, integration, and a sense of progress and continiuty if we do not have the opportunity to work with them consistently over time and if our contacts typically take place in emergency rooms or in a ten-day stay on an inpatient unit, followed by months of no contact.

This is the problem with which we are all struggling as we try to meet the needs of the chronic young adult psychiatric patient. Our community human services networks are facing major difficulties in ensuring not only an adequate level of continuity of care but also the basic conditions of a tolerable life. Once basic needs are met, developing the capacity to provide useful treatment and support emerges as the major mental health challenge of the 1980s.

References

Caton, C. L. M. "The New Chronic Patient and the System of Community Care." *Hospital and Community Psychiatry*, 1981, *32* (7), 475–478.

Goffman, E. *Asylums: Essays on the Social Situation of Mental Patients and Other Inmates*. New York: Doubleday, 1962.

Gruenberg, E. M. "On the Pathogenesis of the Social Breakdown Syndrome." In Mammerborn (Ed.), *A Critical Review of Treatment Progress in a State Hospital Reorganized Toward the Communities Served: Treatment Programs Present and Planned, of the Colorado State Hospital*. Pueblo, Colo.: Colorado State Hospital, 1963, 96–108 (mimeograph).

Gruenberg, E. M. "The Social Breakdown Syndrome and Its Prevention." In G. Caplan (Ed.), *American Handbook of Psychiatry (Volume II): Child and Adolescent Psychiatry, Sociocultural and Community Psychiatry*. (2nd ed.) New York: Basic Books, 1974.

Gruenberg, E. M., Brandon, S., and Kasius, R. V. "Identifying Cases of the Social Breakdown Syndrome." *Milbank Memorial Fund Quarterly*, January 1966 (part 2), *44*, 150–155.

Gruenberg, E. M., Turns, D. M., Segal, S. P., and others. "Social Breakdown Syndrome: Environmental and Host Factors Associated with Chronicity." *American Journal of Public Health*, 1972, *62*, 91–94.

Segal, S. P., and Baumohl, J. "Engaging the Disengaged: Proposals on Madness and Vagrancy." *Social Work*, 1980, *25* (5), 358–365.

Segal, S. P., Baumohl, J., and Johnson, E. "Falling Through the Cracks: Mental Disorder and Social Margin in a Young Vagrant Population." *Social Problems*, 1977, *24* (3), 387–400.

Bert Pepper is a psychiatrist, director of the Rockland County Community Mental Health Center (Pomona, New York), clinical professor of psychiatry at New York University, and chairman of the New York State Conference of Local Mental Hygiene Directors.

Hilary Ryglewicz, ACSW, is clinical assistant to the director at the Rockland County Community Mental Health Center.

Michael C. Kirshner is a psychologist and is director of professional education and training at the Rockland County Community Mental Health Center.

*After a decade of operation, the Hutchings Psychiatric Center
in Syracuse, New York, designed to embrace an acute-care crisis
stabilization model, is characterized by a caseload of young and
chronically disabled individuals.*

The Young Adult Chronic Patient: Three Hypothesized Subgroups

*John L. Sheets
James A. Prevost
Jacqueline Reihman*

As part of the construction program begun by the New York State Department of Mental Hygiene in the mid-1960s, a new breed of state psychiatric hospitals was conceptualized and built, of which Hutchings Psychiatric Center is an example. Hutchings was constructed to serve the Syracuse metropolitan area of 463,000 persons, and later its services were extended to four surrounding counties, now a total population of 770,000. Hutchings' range of services was designed more along the lines of a community mental health center than those of a traditional psychiatric hospital. In its short history, Hutchings has already witnessed continual growth and increasing demands on its staff and services. Specifically, since the turn of the decade, Hutchings has experienced a significant increase in the numbers of people seeking help: from 3,000 in 1979 to 3,600 in 1980, a 20 percent increase over a one-year period. There are various hypotheses to explain the increase in service demands that has occurred both

Adapted from Sheets, J. L., Prevost, J. A., and Reihman, J. "Young Adult Chronic Patients: Three Hypothesized Subgroups." *Hospital and Community Psychiatry*, March 1982, *33*, 197–202.

B. Pepper, H. Ryglewicz (Eds.). *New Directions for Mental Health Services: The Young Adult Chronic Patient*, no. 14. San Francisco: Jossey-Bass, June 1982.

statewide and nationwide. Much of this volume is an attempt to explore and explain these changes. What has become clear is that the single group most demanding of services is the young adult chronic patient. Before services can be developed for the coming decade, it is necessary to define the numbers and characteristics of the young adult chronic population, what their service needs are, and what impact they are having on the current service system.

Defining the Patient

Using a conceptual framework developed by Minkoff (1978) it was found that chronicity may be defined in any of three ways: (1) diagnosis: typically includes organic conditions, schizophrenia, the major affective disorders, and some personality disorders; (2) duration of stay: usually defined as one year or more of hospitalization; and (3) disability: usually defined as an impairment of role performance or daily living function skills. In addition, Goldman, Gattozzi, and Taube (1981) and Wing (1978) have reported that chronicity for long-term patients maintained in the community, at least in terms of functional disability, may also be inferred from the services they use — sheltered workshops, supervised residences, and day programs. Indicators for each of these chronicity criteria were constructed and applied to 2,361 individuals of all ages served by Hutchings in 1979. From this, it was found that 1,232 (or over half of all patients) were judged to be chronic by a combination of diagnosis, duration of stay, and disability criteria.

Since the single largest age group served by Hutchings is that of the young adult eighteen to thirty-four years old, it was hypothesized that a significant proportion of those regarded as chronic would not have been in the system long enough to have been defined chronic with the more traditional diagnosis or duration-of-stay criteria. This was supported when, by eliminating both diagnosis and history of hospitalization, it was found that 966, or 41 percent of the Hutchings 1979 population, could be described as chronic by functional disability alone. Further, of those 966 persons judged chronic by functional disability, 369, or 36 percent, were between the ages of eighteen and thirty-four.

The Typical Chronic Young Adult Patient

To clarify the clinical and demographic characteristics of the young adult patients at Hutchings, a statistical description of the average young adult patient in 1979 was developed and compared with similar profiles for older chronic patients. From this composite, the young chronically disabled adult at Hutchings is typified as a single white male, age twenty-seven, who lives in the city of Syracuse, as opposed to in the suburbs. He is first admitted to Hutchings on an involuntary basis when he is twenty-two years of age and receives a diagnosis of schizophrenia. Since then, he is hospitalized slightly less than once a year. When he is hospitalized each year, it is usually for a short stay averaging less than thirty days. Since his first inpatient admission three years ago, he has been admitted or transferred five times between inpatient, outpatient, and day treatment services. During 1979, he received both inpatient and outpatient services and, in addition, he used either a supervised residence or a supervised day program. As of January, 1980, he is still being actively followed by a Hutchings service.

If we were to compare the young adult chronic patient with the middle-aged chronic patient at Hutchings, the profile is similar, except that the middle-aged person is a forty-nine-year-old woman who enters the system for the first time when she is forty-three, and since that time is hospitalized slightly less than once every two years. In 1979, she used only outpatient services and, like her young adult counterpart, as of July, 1980, she is still active in the system.

Community Functioning of Patients

To develop a perspective on the community functioning of young adult chronic patients at Hutchings, data were referenced which enabled a comparison of the community functioning of eighteen- to thirty-five-year-olds with those thirty-six and older. Figure 1 shows the domains of functioning which were assessed and the percentages of persons in each age group who reported having difficulties in the domain. Aside from the physical disabilities category and the personal hygiene domain, the group eighteen to thirty-five consistently displayed greater difficulty in navigating community life situations than the older chronic population.

Treatment Histories

The treatment careers of the 369 young adult chronic patients identified in 1979 were reviewed at four different points in time over twenty-two months. At all sample points, nearly 60 percent of this patient population was receiving some type of inpatient, outpatient, or day treatment service. It was

Figure 1. Community Functioning Problems of Hutchings Community Support Services (CSS) Clients

Community Functioning Domain	Percent of Patients Reporting Problems 18–35 Years	36 + Years
Physical Disabilities	45%	70%
Personal Hygiene	31%	35%
Psychiatric Symptoms	47%	20%
Daily Living Skills	66%	53%
Behavior Problems	35%	8%
Social Isolation	73%	59%
Alcohol, Drug Abuse	25%	11%

also found that a core group of 124 (or 34 percent) of the original 369 were enrolled in service on all sample dates. Further review indicated that in addition to the 34 percent who were found to be present on all four dates, 49 percent were intermittently enrolled in service over the twenty-two months, and 17 percent were not enrolled at all.

In order to further examine the characteristics of these young adult patients, a systematic sample of fifty of the persons actively enrolled in Hutchings programs in May 1981 was compared with a sample of fifty-five of those not active on any of the four previous dates. It is important to note that the sample of fifty active in May 1981 is made up of a combination of those who were active on all four dates and those who were enrolled intermittently.

The median age differed by only one year for the enrolled and not enrolled groups, twenty-six and twenty-seven years respectively. Similarly, the groups were evenly distributed with regard to gender with both groups showing a slight predominance of men: 58 percent for those enrolled and 53 percent for those not enrolled. In examining the dimension of ethnicity, though, an association was detected between 'group' and ethnic status, with the enrolled group showing 20 percent black and the not enrolled showing 7 percent. [Association between 'group' and ethnic status: $(X_3^2 = 4.60; p < .10)$.] Of the other variables examined, the most dramatic differences were found in diagnoses. A significant relationship was found between enrollment status and the presence or absence of a schizophrenic diagnosis. [Association between 'enrolled' group and schizophrenic diagnosis: $(X_3^2 = 11.21; p < .001)$.] Specifically, only 25 percent of those persons not enrolled in any services were diagnosed as schizophrenic while a full 64 percent of those actively enrolled were. This latter percentage is also significantly different from the 25 percent diagnosed schizophrenic in the age group eighteen to thirty-four.

Since the fifty-five persons in the not enrolled category were no longer HPC patients, it was not possible to secure additional information about them. However, it was possible to obtain additional data for the fifty persons still utilizing HPC services. Their profiles may be characterized by the following: 90 percent of these persons are unmarried, over 75 percent are unemployed and/or receive either Public Assistance or SSI (Supplemental Security Income), and over 80 percent currently use psychotropic drugs. Nearly half of these persons have completed high school and two thirds live in their own home or apartment, either alone or with family or spouse. This finding is similar to that reported by Lamb and Goertzel (1977) which showed that, contrary to popular belief, less than a third of young and chronically disabled individuals in this era of community treatment live in board-and-care homes or cheap hotels. Most, they indicate, live in nonsegregated, noninstitutional settings.

Finally, over half of the sample of fifty first entered the Hutchings system when they were between the ages of thirteen and twenty and 22 percent were found to be developmentally disabled.

Figure 2. Hypothesized Typology of
Young Adult Chronic Patients

System-Dependent Group	High-Energy/High-Demand Group	High-Functioning Group
Most probably began mental health involvement in early adolescence	Able to shop around from agency to agency to get what they want	Generally higher S.E.S. (socioeconomic status) and better appearance
Firmly ensconced in role of patient	Changing functional abilities and interests	New to mental health system
Do not do well, even in remission	"Give me what I want or stay out of my life" attitude toward mental health	Resistant to mental health program involvement on the basis of conviction
Concretely attached to specific programs and program places	Low frustration tolerance, acting out, encounters with the law	Some entered mental health system via alcoholism or drug abuse
Passive, poorly motivated	Frequently evicted, mobile	Want to understand their disorders and ways of preventing future breakdowns
Accepting of mental health services	Expectations for making it on their own	
Appear burned out at an early age	Includes "revolving-door" repeaters and street people	Want to blend into general population without being identified as mental patients

Young Adult Subgroups

In a related but independent effort, data was sought which would illuminate the personal behavior of young adult chronic patients and what one would likely experience in a service encounter with them. To achieve this, twenty-two key informants from state, county, and voluntary agencies were interviewed.

The single most profound theme which surfaced from these interviews is that young adults with chronic disabilities, while they have youth and loneliness in common, are not all alike; in fact, they can be dramatically different from one another. Further, the factors which apparently account for these differences include developmental stage, functional ability, socioeconomic background, and life style.

A content analysis of interviews allowed us to identify both similarities and differences in young chronic patients. From this analysis three distinct groups of patients emerged, each with identifiable characteristics, and each with a full complement of service needs and wants. These groups, summarized in Figure 2, include the following.

The Low Energy, Low Demand Group. This group likely entered a state hospital or state school setting as a child or adolescent and, hence, is already well ensconced in the role of patienthood and is characterized by passivity and low motivation.

The High Energy, High Demand Group. This is the group that generates groans and cries in case managers. When they want something, either money, discharge papers, or you (their therapist), they want it right away! And when they don't want you or your services, they want you to leave them alone. When they feel ignored or neglected, they have the mobility and confronting skills to shop around. Their low tolerance for frustration and impulsive behaviors frequently result in encounters with the law. Impulsivity often culminates in eviction, and they often end up in the streets.

Compounding this, physical mobility produces financial instability. SSI and Public Assistance checks are often held up or terminated when these patients move without notice. They may lose their Public Assistance eligibility by taking a job at Burger King for two days and then leaving after an explosive encounter with the manager.

These patients are not without aspirations; they have bought America's Madison Avenue campaigns and spend their limited funds on TVs, stereos, and tape decks. Possessing few sexual inhibitions, they meet one another on inpatient units, fall in love, and bear children. But because of their unstable life styles, their children are most often placed permanently in foster care.

The High Functioning, High Aspiration Group. This is a group typified by the ability to function much of the time at a fairly high level. Many have more education and are more attractive than the average patient. But their appearance can be misleading; these patients are or have been seriously disabled by their disorders and are often without social support. Yet they find planned mental activities demeaning. They do not want to be identified with traditional mental health programs, older chronic patients, or with age peers who are more debilitated than themselves. This group actively seeks information and expresses neither hopelessness nor helplessness about their disorders; indeed, they feel very keenly the expectations of their families, their staff, and themselves, and they hold out hope for fulfillment of these expectations. What they want most of all is the opportunity to blend into the general population to see if they can pass. (The description of this hypothesized subgroup is derived from an unpublished Report on Psychosocial Rehabilitation Programs submitted to the Title XX Training Unit of the New York State Office of Mental Health in September, 1979 by Sheila LeGacy of Transitional Living Services, Inc. and Edward Benson of Hutchings Psychiatric Center in Syracuse, New York).

Data Comparisons

The data reported to this point are derived from different methodologies and hence are not directly comparable. It is, however, instructive to review their qualitative similarities. Specifically, you will note the striking congruence which exists between the characteristics of the random sample of fifty young adults enrolled in service on all four sample dates and of the hypothesized system-dependent group. These sampled patients are dependent consumers of services who by and large entered the service system as adolescents.

Because of the limited nature of the data, we are unable to make specific statements regarding the congruence between the hypothesized high functioning group and the sample of patients not enrolled in any HPC service. Some speculation, however, is warranted. It was argued that the high functioning group would function relatively well in remission, a notion supported by the less severe diagnoses assigned to the not enrolled sample. In the absence of hard data addressing reasons for the sample groups' nonparticipation in HPC services, it seems logical to argue that they may well believe traditional mental health services to be demeaning.

Finally, although no empirical data have yet been assembled which provide support for the hypothesized high energy, high demand group, a report by Schwartz and Goldfinger (1981) supporting the existence of this subgroup and qualitative evidence for the other two components of the typology is certainly strong enough to warrant increased attention.

As a whole, these findings suggest that we should pursue more rigorously the notion of the taxonomy given the fact that services and styles of relating to the subgroups may need to vary in order for interventions to be effective. Whereas the system dependent group may need and accept traditional bench assembly sheltered work, for example, the high functioning group would most likely reject it in favor of the more creative vocational programs, such as transitional employment placements or employment in a restaurant operating under a vocational evaluation and training certificate. Also, whereas the most dependent group is likely to accept psycho-social clubs, which operate from a single location, the higher functioning group would likely require clubs without walls — networks of people and activities which occur in a variety of community settings including homes, restaurants, and neighborhood pubs. For the erratic group there may be a need for youth oriented drop-in centers, temporary shelters, and day labor vocational alternatives.

Conclusions for Designing Services

Although a precise picture of the characteristics and needs of the young adult chronic population is still being formulated, the problems, aspirations, and demands of the group are already challenging our conventional wisdom. In response to this challenge, we will need to think and respond differently in the way we plan and provide treatment, rehabilitation, and community support services.

Some of the changes that are required include the following: First, there is a need to make better use of epidemiological and demographic predictive methods in the planning of mental health systems. This is required to know how many people in specific age groups with particular problems will need specific types of services. Second, we need to realistically include indefinite term inpatient and indefinite term community residence options in the array of services defining a comprehensive mental health system. This is to accommodate those patients who do not respond totally to acute care models of service and who, therefore, require special health care, protective custody, and security control devices. Third, through education and training there is a need to reorient mental health professionals and paraprofessionals to the principles and practices of chronic care, specifically how it differs from acute care models of service. It would be essential to convey, for example, that the treatment values of transcendance, independence, normalization, and cure may be inappropriate myths when unrealistically applied to chronic patients. Fourth, there is a need to be more precise in understanding and acknowledging the total range of needs of the chronically disabled to enable prescriptive and targeted provision of services. It will be necessary to accept with hope rather than despair the limits of treatment and the realistic expectations of rehabilitation and indefinite term community support services. Fifth, there is a need to design programs which are more age, culture, and disability level specific such as drop-in centers for the young and senior citizen club programs for the aged. Sixth, there is a need to adapt our interpersonal clinical styles of relating to this population and to become more willing to enter life's enterprise with them. And, seventh, assuming we are entering a new era and will make mistakes along the way, we need to establish our programs in a way that implicitly includes evaluation of them. It is only by developing this data based information that we can look back years from now and accurately assess the impact of our services on the disorder, the duration of stay, the life functioning, and the life satisfaction of this group.

References

Cotton, P. G., Bene-Kocemba, A., and Cole, R. "The Effect of Deinstitutionalization on a General Hospital's Psychiatric Unit." *Hospital and Community Psychiatry,* 1979, *30,* 609–612.

Goldman, H., Gattozzi, A. A., and Taube, C. A. "Defining and Counting the Chronically Mentally Ill." *Hospital and Community Psychiatry,* 1981, *32,* 21–25.

Kramer, M. "Population Changes and Schizophrenia 1970–1985." Paper presented at the Second Rochester International Conference on Schizophrenia, Rochester, New York, May 1976.

Lamb, H. R., and Goertzel, V. "The Long-Term Patient in the Era of Community Treatment." *Archives of General Psychiatry*, 1977, *34*, 679-682.

Minkoff, K. "A Map of Chronic Patients." In J. A. Talbott (Ed.), *The Chronic Mental Patient*. Washington, D.C.: American Psychiatric Association, 1978.

Pepper, B., Kirshner, M., and Ryglewicz, H. "The Young Adult Chronic Patient: Overview of a Population." *Hospital and Community Psychiatry*, 1981, *32*, 463-469.

Pepper, B., and Ryglewicz, H. "The Young Adult Chronic Patient. Keynote Address: Overview of the Population and the Issues." Paper presented at the Conference on The Young Adult Chronic Patient, Suffern, New York, November 20-21, 1980.

Schwartz, S., and Goldfinger, S. "The New Chronic Patient: Clinical Characteristics of an Emerging Subgroup." *Hospital and Community Psychiatry*, 1981, *32*, 470-474.

Shore, M. F., and Shapiro, R. "The Effects of Deinstitutionalization on the State Hospital." *Hospital and Community Psychiatry*, 1979, *30*, 605-608.

Wing, J. K. "Who Becomes Chronic." *Psychiatric Quarterly*, 1978, *50* (3), 179-190.

John L. Sheets is director of rehabilitation services at Hutchings Psychiatric Center, and Jacqueline Reihman is director of program evaluation at the same institution. Both are assistant professors of psychiatry at the State University of New York (SUNY) Upstate Medical Center in Syracuse, New York. James A. Prevost is commissioner, New York State Office of Mental Health and formerly the director of Hutchings; he is also a professor of psychiatry at SUNY, Upstate Medical Center.

The impact of the size and nature of the young adult patient
population on the general hospital system is illustrated
by recent research reports.

Serving the Young Adult
Chronic Patient in the 1980s:
Challenge to the General Hospital

Gladys Egri
Carol L. M. Caton

Why is it that the young adult chronic patient is a topic today and has been one of the most talked-about issues for at least the past year among mental health professionals working in the public sector? These young adult patients represent the same diagnostic groups as their elders: they react equally to medication, and they struggle, like every generation, to master the life crises of young adulthood. Still, despite our more refined diagnostic schemes and the larger repertoire of pharmacologic treatments, we frequently fail either to affect the course of their illness or to improve the quality of their lives. This failure poses a serious threat to our sense of professional competence and challenges our commitment to serve the communities in which we are located. There is a growing number of reports in the literature describing the unique characteristics of young adult chronic patients in various locales, in different types of mental health delivery systems. The most common characteristics of troublesome young adult patients are their serious deficits in coping and adaptation abilities. The socially disturbing behavior of the young adult patient, coupled with noncompliance and misuse of existing treatments, poses critical

B. Pepper, H. Ryglewicz (Eds.). *New Directions for Mental Health Services: The Young Adult Chronic Patient*, no. 14. San Francisco: Jossey-Bass, June 1982.

25

problems to the community and to components of the mental health delivery system, including the general hospital.

All service systems are encountering an increased number of patients who are under thirty-five years of age. As Bachrach (1981) has pointed out, there are at least two major factors that are accountable for such an increase. First, deinstitutionalization and related policies produced large numbers of patients who reside in communities; prior to this era, they would have spent great proportions of their lives in hospitals. Second, there is a shift in the demographic composition of the nation; one-third of the population, or about 64 million persons are between twenty and thirty-four years of age—the age group that is at major risk of developing schizophrenia and manic depressive disorder.

These two factors create a variety of different demands on hospitals. The already chronic group requires mainly tertiary intervention to minimize their disability. The recently ill, but not yet chronic, requires early diagnosis and adequate treatment to minimize the risk of development of chronic disability. Both groups of patients will increase in size during the next decade, due to the cohort increases (Bachrach, 1981). Descriptive studies of these groups have been appearing in recent years in the literature. Segal and others (1977) studied young vagrants in Berkeley, California in 1973. They found that 22 percent of them had histories of mental illness. Robbins and others (1978) studied the hospital charts of a group of inpatients at Bellevue Hospital in New York City, considered by staff to have received "maximum hospital benefit." (Staff no longer wanted to treat them.) Typically, these patients are young men with few social or vocational skills who respond to stress with rage, augmented by alcoholism or drug abuse. A study conducted by Pepper and others at a Community Mental Health Center in Rockland County, New York, was reported among other studies in the July 1981 issue of *Hospital and Community Psychiatry* (Pepper and Ryglewicz, 1980; Pepper, Kirshner, and Ryglewicz, 1981). In a similar study of young adults seen at a comprehensive State hospital in Upstate New York in a one-year period, Sheets (1981) obtained comparable data. In both cases close to half had three or more inpatient admissions. Also alcohol and drug abuse were a significant factor in the disability of both groups.

The studies conducted by Segal, Robbins, Sheets, and Pepper covered different geographic areas, different types of delivery systems, and different ethnic and social groups. All these studies identified subgroups of young adult chronic patients presenting specific problems to the mental health system, and they suggest the need to further define the subgroups contained in this population. For example, the group described by Robbins is in striking contrast to the group described by Segal. Berkeley's vagrants perceived themselves not as ill but as poor social outcasts who considered the hospital as an equivalent to jail in which their freedom was lost along with the last vestige of their autonomy and self esteem. The Bellevue patients, on the other hand, presented themselves as sick and dependent and expected the hospital to provide long-term nurturance and support in all areas of life.

Characteristics which define other subgroups include suicide potential (Caton, 1981),* criminal acting out, and inability to care for dependent children. It should be noted that patients in this age group are in their reproductive years and have opportunities for procreation which did not exist in the era of the asylum. Thus, we find that the behavior of troublesome young adult patients touches many lives and can be unpleasant at best and very destructive or dangerous at its worst.

The General Hospital System and the Young Adult Chronic Patient

The general hospital has become one of the most important facilities in the care of the mentally ill as it has been taking over the bulk of inpatient care. The number of units has grown from under forty in the 1940s to 940 in 1974. With the increase of numbers of units, the number of patients and the types of services have increased as well. General hospital psychiatric departments now include a range of programs from emergency room to inpatient care to outpatient community programs.

Over the past twenty years, the general hospital has assumed increasing responsibility for the chronic and seriously impaired patient to such an extent that it is now the major provider of psychiatric care for this group; it is predicted to become the core service to succeed the state hospital (Greenhill, 1979). Concomitantly, the general hospital is frequently the recipient of the communities' problems and the caretaker of its health. All problems that affect the lives of the residents of the area in which it is located influence the demand for services by the hospital.

The impact of the size and nature of the young adult patient population on the general hospital system is illustrated by recent research reports. A longitudinal study of psychiatric emergency room utilization over a two decade period in New Haven, Connecticut (Bristol, Giller, and Docharty, 1981), revealed a shift toward greater numbers of young, single, nonwhite males. This study also found an increase in both schizophrenia and alcoholism among the young. It was concluded that young males suffered from more severe disorders, based on their higher hospitalization rates. In a recent study of the new type of chronic patients in a San Francisco general hospital emergency room, the most problematic patients were found to be predominantly male, single, and transient; these patients had serious ego deficits, few skills, and no social

---

*The referenced study by Carol L. M. Caton reported, for a New York City cohort of 119 patients, five successful suicides within a follow-up period of one year. Unpublished results of follow-up over a longer period indicated an even higher suicide rate, concentrated in the lower portion of the eighteen to thirty age group of young adult males.

supports ("New York City Community Support System Monitoring and Evaluation Report," 1981). A study of eleven New York City municipal hospitals revealed that the modal age of patients admitted to their emergency rooms and inpatient units was in the early twenties (Schwartz and Goldfinger, 1981).

Harlem Hospital is one of the eleven New York City municipal hospitals studied. A review of all patients admitted to the psychiatric emergency room in October 1980, revealed that during that month a total of 197 patients were seen. About 60 percent of the total group were males, primarily under thirty-five years of age. Nearly half of this group had a primary diagnosis of schizophrenia; the second most common diagnosis was alcoholism and drug abuse. In contrast, females under thirty-five were equally divided in the schizophrenia and major affective disorder categories. Many patients had multiple diagnoses. Several had return emergency room visits during that period. A small number currently lived outside of the Harlem area, although most had their roots in Harlem. Those few categorized as undomiciled were squatters in abandoned buildings. It is notable that similar sex and diagnostic characteristics existed for program attendees at Harlem Rehabilitation Center, a comprehensive social and vocational community-based rehabilitation arm of Harlem Hospital Center, as for emergency room presentees.

A three-year follow-up review of the 121 patients (Egri, 1981) admitted in 1976 showed that their functional outcome (as defined by performing an expected societal role; either as student, worker, or homemaker) was not determined by either age, sex, diagnosis, or number of prior hospitalizations. The only predictor of good outcome was "graduation" from the Harlem Rehabilitation Center program — that is, termination by mutual agreement between staff and patient. About 60 percent fell into this category. For those who "graduated" 75 percent did well for three years.

While an equal proportion of all groups "graduated," there was an age and sex difference among those who did not complete their program successfully. Those for whom services were terminated due to disruptive behavior and substance abuse were concentrated in the under-twenty-five-year-old male group.

The number of troublesome young patients has been increasing and is continuing to increase in the unit. Changes have been instituted in the content of the program to make it more relevant to their interests; more intensive personal liaison has been developed with referring agencies to facilitate patients' engagement in the program. Still, violent outbursts are more frequent than in the past. Both staff and the older patients find many of these patients' attitudes and behavior to be detrimental to the total community's activities and development and to be highly taxing their time and energies. There is also an increasing number of young people, mainly males, whose institutional experience is shared equally between psychiatric hospitals and prison. In their search for long-term asylum, they almost consciously commit criminal acts in a manner that will assure them total care, which at present is available only in the penitentiary.

It is our impression that the factors that were most influential in both compliance with treatment plans and eventual functional improvement were personality attributes of the patients, rather than diagnosis, length of illness or number of prior hospitalizations. Frustration tolerance, quality of judgment, ability to plan toward a goal, ability to delay gratification, toleration of stress without resorting to the use of psychoactive substances or acting-out are among the most important attributes. Most patients who possessed enough ego resources to at least start in the program, had the potential to grow, change their behavior and develop a healthier self-concept and more mature interpersonal relationships.

What Goes Wrong in Treatment of the Young Adult Patient? Rehabilitation components of units in general hospitals are more the exception than the rule. Few hospitals have the opportunity to learn first-hand about the changing disabilities of their patients. Periodic review of emergency room utilization patterns has been recommended as a tool for better service planning (Bristol, Giller, and Docharty, 1981). In the light of our present knowledge, it appears that there are a host of factors contributing to the frequent failure to affect positively the lives of these patients once they are in contact with the hospital. Prominently significant are the sites in which evaluation and treatment are provided; the patients' unattractive appearance and intractable behavior; the negative attitude of the staff towards them; funding and other regulatory constraints imposed on the units; environmental and social factors outside of the influence of the hospital; inadequate models for diagnosis and treatment. In addition, those patients who do not consider themselves sick and who resent having to deal with hospitals and the establishment as a whole arrive with the most negative attitude, which challenges our aptitude to change hostility and negativism to cooperation and trust.

In addition, some characteristics of specific service programs can be obstacles. The emergency room, which is the usual portal of entry into the general hospital system of care is usually frantic and overcrowded and cannot usually support the time and effort required to conduct a comprehensive diagnosis and the development of a treatment contract. It is often staffed by trainees and junior staff whose lack of experience can result in more frequent use of the inpatient service as the easiest disposition (Feigelson, Davis, and McKinnon, 1978). The inpatient services, for their part, are typically directed toward short-stay, acute care. The treatment goal is that of rapid control of symptoms; utilization of regulations and reimbursement formulas that are based on standards developed by the other departments of the hospital constrain the ability to base length of stay on all relevant clinical criteria (Bachrach, 1981). Legal issues, such as the right to treatment and the right to refuse treatment also pose obstacles to effective treatment delivery.

Establishment of a therapeutic alliance is a key factor for adequate diagnosis and effective treatment. There is an array of reasons and circumstances that make such an alliance difficult to establish with these patients. Concordance of goals between patient and physician has been found to predict the patient's likelihood of following up on recommended treatment (Jellinek, 1978). The goals of young adult chronic patients and those of the mental health professional are often discordant.

Because many of these patients' problems lie outside what is covered by our present diagnostic schemes, our present methods of evaluation only describe a part of the clinical picture they present, leaving many of the significant elements unidentified, undescribed, and unresolved. The reductionist "rule-out" technique of the biomedical model in use does not consider all the personal attributes patients have. The inadequacy of this model in medicine as a whole and in psychiatry in particular has been pointed out for some time. Several authors have called for the substitution of this way of approaching diagnosis and treatment by a biopsychosocial model that would allow for a broad consideration of the person as a whole.

Diagnostic difficulties exist also because so many of these patients arrive at the emergency room in varied stages of intoxication that mask other symptoms of an underlying disorder. Their mistrust of authority and their style of communication make the medical histories they give unreliable.

What Can Hospitals Do About the Chronic Young Adult Patient? The drawbacks of not having a mental health system with delimited responsibilities for target groups and specific service types are dramatically illustrated by these patients. Because of the multiplicity of problems they present, only a concerted effort and a combination of systems can have positive results.

The magnitude and nature of problems created and experienced by young adult patients varies from one area to another. It is impossible to generalize these patients' characteristics or to refer to the general hospital system as a whole. In other words, there is no typical general hospital patient. Careful studies of categories of young adult patients are needed, based on a comprehensive appraisal of their problems and personal attributes. Such studies in turn can facilitate better crisis intervention and development of treatment plans as well as broadening the skills of mental health professionals in the public sector. They will also provide data necessary to recommend development of programs by other human service systems, which ought to complement hospital services. It is already apparent that patients' needs range from long-term hospitalization, to drop-in crisis treatment and socialization programs as well as a range of educational, training, and employment opportunities and a range of supportive living facilities. Each subgroup requires quite different services.

Because its helping hand extends far into the community, the general hospital can feel the pulse beat of its constituency at large. Each hospital can assess the unique needs of its people, document it through data collection, and attempt to influence public policies and funding mechanisms to respond most effectively to this major public health issue of the 1980s.

References

Bachrach, L. L. "Planning Mental Health Services for Chronic Patients." *Hospital and Community Psychiatry*, 1979, *30*, 387–393.

Bachrach, L. L. "Program Planning for Young Adult Chronic Patients." Paper presented at the Conference on The Young Adult Chronic Patient II, Albany, N.Y., June 1981.

Bachrach, L. L. "General Hospital Psychiatry: Overview from a Sociological Perspective." *American Journal of Psychiatry,* 1981, *138,* 879–887.

Bristol, J. H., Giller, E., and Docharty, J. P. "Trends in Emergency Psychiatry in the Last Two Decades." *American Journal of Psychiatry,* 1981, *138,* 623–628.

Caton, C. L. M. "The New Chronic Patient and the System of Community Care." *Hospital and Community Psychiatry,* 1981, *32* (7), 475–478.

Egri, G. "Psychiatric Rehabilitation in Harlem: A Three-Year Follow-up of 121 Chronic Patients." Presented at St. Lukes-Roosevelt Hospital Center's Grand Rounds, January 1981.

Engel, G. L. "The Need for a New Medical Model: A Challenge for Biomedicine." *Science,* 1977, *196,* 129–136.

Feigelson, E. B., Davis, E. B., McKinnon, R., and others. "The Decision to Hospitalize." *American Journal of Psychiatry,* 1978, *135,* 354–357.

Flamm, G. H. "The Expanding Roles of General-Hospital Psychiatry." *Hospital and Community Psychiatry,* 1979, *30,* 190–192.

Gerson, S., and Bassuk, E. L. "Psychiatric Emergencies: An Overview." *American Journal of Psychiatry,* 1980, *137,* 1–11.

Greenhill, M. H. "Psychiatric Units in General Hospitals: 1979." *Hospital and Community Psychiatry,* 1979, *30,* 109–182.

Jellinek, M. "Referrals from a Psychiatric Emergency Room: Relationship of Compliance to Demographic and Interview Variables." *American Journal of Psychiatry,* 1978, *135,* 209–213.

"New York City Community Support System Monitoring and Evaluation Report." June 1981.

Pepper, B., Kirshner, M., and Ryglewicz, H. "The Young Adult Chronic Patient: Overview of a Population." *Hospital and Community Psychiatry,* 1981, *32,* 463–469.

Pepper, B., and Ryglewicz, H. "The Young Adult Chronic Patient: Keynote Address: Overview of the Population and the Issues." Presented at the Conference on the Young Adult Chronic Patient, Suffern, N.Y., November 1980.

Robbins, E., Stern, M., Robbin, L., and others. "Unwelcome Patients: Where Can They Find Asylum?" *Hospital and Community Psychiatry,* 1978, *24,* 44–46.

Schwartz, S. R., and Goldfinger, S. M. "The New Chronic Patient: Clinical Characteristics of an Emerging Subgroup." *Hospital and Community Psychiatry,* 1981, *32,* 470–474.

Segal, S. P., Baumohl, J., and Johnson, E. "Falling Through the Cracks: Mental Disorder and Social Margin in a Young Vagrant Population." *Social Problems,* 1977, *24,* 387–400.

Sheets, J. L. "Current Profiles of the Young Adult Chronic Patient at Hutchings Psychiatric Center, Syracuse, New York." Presented at The Young Adult Chronic Patient II: A Conference on the Major Mental Health Challenge for the 1980s. Albany, N.Y., June 3–5, 1981.

Gladys Egri is a psychiatrist and chief, Partial Hospitalization Program, Psychiatry Service, VA Medical Center, Buffalo, New York, and clinical associate professor of psychiatry, State University of New York, Buffalo, and lecturer in psychiatry, Columbia University.

Carol L. M. Caton is assistant professor, department of psychiatry, College of Physicians and Surgeons, Columbia University.

Studies show a radical transformation in the ranks and numbers of the homeless, now including large numbers of young, severely disturbed and disabled street people. Without decent, safe, accessible shelter, therapeutic efforts are doomed.

Not Making It Crazy: The Young Homeless Patients in New York City

Kim Hopper
Ellen Baxter
Stuart Cox

If accounts in the popular press are to be believed, a spectre is haunting New York City—the spectre of homelessness. According to official figures, an estimated 36,000 men and women are thought to be periodically or permanently homeless (Office of Mental Health, 1979; Manhattan Bowery Corporation, 1979), at a time when public and private shelters together can accommodate at most 4,200 persons. As a result, thousands ride the subways all night; hundreds try to pass the late hours undetected in train or bus depots; others huddle in doorways or camp out in abandoned buildings; still others haunt the public parks, loading docks in commercial districts, or piers along the rivers. Many walk all night, preferring to snatch what sleep they can in public places in the daytime (Baxter and Hopper, 1981).

In critical respects, this appears to be a new phenomenon. True, large urban centers have always known the homeless—the vagabonds, hoboes, and derelicts who made up the armies of casual labor and populated the legendary skid rows (Anderson, 1923; Bahr, 1970; Bendiner, 1961; Kromer, 1935; Wal-

B. Pepper, H. Ryglewicz (Eds.). *New Directions for Mental Health Services: The Young Adult Chronic Patient*, no. 14. San Francisco: Jossey-Bass, June 1982.

lace, 1965). But the past decade has seen a radical transformation in the ranks and numbers of the homeless. Women now appear in growing numbers; men under forty currently comprise the majority of the Bowery's population; chronic alcoholism is no longer the dominant scourge of the homeless, if it ever was (see Bahr, 1973, p. 103); and the presence of large numbers of severely disturbed and disabled street people is obvious to even the most casual passerby.

Mental health officials have not been oblivious to the crisis. The regional director of the State's Office of Mental Health recently characterized homelessness as "the single greatest problem in New York City today" (*New York Times,* 1981). Recognition of the problem, however, rarely translates into acknowledgment of the role that past mental health policy has played in exacerbating the problem of homelessness and in shaping public attitudes toward it. Roughly half of the city's homeless poor are thought to be mentally disabled, many of them former residents of state psychiatric facilities (Office of Mental Health, 1979; Reich and Siegel, 1978). Nobody knows for sure how many there are, for the simple reason that most of these individuals have long since been lost to service providers. But the sources of their disaffiliation are not difficult to trace. For much of the fourteen year history of intensive deinstitutionalization, inadequate discharge planning, weak follow-up efforts, and scarce supportive housing were the rule (Baxter and Hopper, 1980). When combined with rampant inflation, rising rents, fixed subsistence incomes, and a shrinking supply of low-income dwellings, these factors virtually ensured a swelling of the ranks of the homeless.

Mental health authorities are sometimes wont to respond that the aftercare situation has been rectified and that careful planning for placement outside the hospital is now standard practice (Haveliwala, 1981). Recent data renders the claim suspect. A report from the Office of Mental Health, dated March 31, 1980, details the performance of the state psychiatric centers in discharging patients during fiscal year 1979–1980. In that year, 1,851 releases from such facilities (23 percent) were to "unknown" living arrangements. In one hospital, the proportion of "unknowns" among discharges reached an astonishing 59 percent. Clerical oversight aside, surely many of these destinations were unknown because the patients had no place to go. Moreover, even were the claim substantiated, the response would miss the point: the dam broke more than a decade ago, and relief efforts are only now getting under way.

In what follows, we will address the specific circumstances of one subgroup of the homeless: the young, psychiatrically disabled population. Our focus on this group implies no forgetfulness of the plight of older chronic patients but merely acknowledges the subject of this volume.

The Legacy of the Revolving Door

In 1973, as the first reports on the effects of deinstitutionalization began to appear, Robert Reich described the plight of expatients as "a national disgrace" (1973, p. 1). Six years later, John Talbott simply added an adverb in updating the picture of the chronically mentally ill: "still a national disgrace" (1979, p. 1). Despite the achievements of a few federal demonstration projects (Estroff, 1981; Polak and Kirby, 1976; Rubin, 1980; Test and Stein, 1976), few observers would disagree that the dismal situation persists. Recently, concern has mounted over the prospects of a new cohort of young chronic patients. Veterans of the revolving door trade, the mentally disabled under thirty-five have emerged as the problem patients of the 1980s. They confound conventional treatment efforts, place undue demands on emergency services, resist attempts to engage them in rehabilitation programs, and exhaust the energy and resources of community mental health workers (Pepper and others, 1981; Schwartz and Goldfinger, 1981). Ties with friends and family members are badly frayed where they exist at all. As a result, their lives outside the clinic are typically bereft of the usual sources of support needed in times of distress (Chafetz and Terry, 1981). Among those who are disabled, disaffiliated, the literally homeless, bizarre behavior and unpredictability compound the hardships of street survival, producing a separate class — the so-called space cases. Their transience, the chronicity of their affliction, the fact that available services are ill-suited to their needs, community fear of and distaste for their numbers, and their alleged propensity for violence all conspire to keep them beyond the pale of traditional outreach measures (Segal and Baumohl, 1980; Segal and others, 1977). Nor should the hazards of a marginal existence in the community be underestimated. One study of 119 new chronic patients discharged after short hospital stays and referred to aftercare clinics, reported an astonishing 4.2 percent suicide rate (Caton, 1981). That the clinical predicament is little short of desperate is evident in the plaint of one group of practitioners that the young, rootless expatients have "become, individually and collectively, our albatross" (Pepper and others, 1981, p. 464).

The Men We Lodge — Revisited

In March 1914, the Advisory Social Service Committee of the Municipal Lodging House of New York City undertook an investigation of some 2,000 men housed in the Municipal Lodging House. That the subject of their study is not unfamiliar to city dwellers or sociologists today is evident from their opening description: "Withdrawn from the activities and responsibilities of a normal life, he is not unlike many men who, living in hotels, clubs, and boarding houses, might in the strict sense of the word, be called homeless. From these he differs, however, in that his loneliness is often accompanied either by unemployment, or by a complexity of disabilities which make him unemployable. He is not only homeless, but is often without food, shelter or money, and in most cases, if a worker at all, he is a casual worker" (1915, p. 9).

Although a substantial proportion of the men examined were considered unemployable — 11 percent due to physical handicap, at least thirty-nine percent due to alcoholism (it is clear from the text that these percentages overlap)—it is noteworthy that only 10 percent were referred to the Clearing House for Mental Defectives for further clinical attention.

Recall, of course, that this was still the era of the great confinement in state facilities for the insane. The functions of asylum and custody were tightly linked and access so controlled that such facilities provided "a convenient way to get rid of inconvenient people" (Scull, 1977, p. 33). As a result, apparently few chronically mentally disabled people were found among the wandering poor.

How different the situation is today may be gauged from the results of a similar survey conducted sixty-four years after the Advisory Committee's pioneering effort. In May of 1980, the Health Services System (a private agency) and City Human Resources Administration examined some 240 men lodged in one of the city's shelters (on Wards Island). The screening, which extended over three days, paid special attention to the psychiatric condition of the residents. The study found the majority of men in this sample to be in poor mental health. Fully 70 percent of the men were thought to be mentally disordered to some degree; 60 percent of them, moderately or severely so. Sixteen were found in need of immediate hospitalization.

Of particular interest for our purposes here, was the mental health status of the eighty-five residents (35 percent) who were thirty-five years old or younger. Interviews were obtained for eighty of these men. Table 1 summarizes the findings of these examinations. As shown, over two thirds of the younger population was considered to be moderately or severely psychiatrically disabled. Fully 34 percent of them admitted to past hospitalization. Some indication of the degree of disability entailed by the label *moderate* may be

Table 1. Distribution of Disability for Keener Residents Thirty-Five Years or Younger

Degree of Disability*	Number	Percentage
None	15	18.75%
Mild	11	13.75%
Moderate	22	27.5%
Severe	32	40%
Total	80	100%

Note: Categories derived from interviewer rating of overall severity of illness. Prototypical symptoms noted in support of clinical judgments include the following:
Mild—"schizoid tendencies"; "slight delusions of grandeur"; mild depression and anxiety; past hospitalization
Moderate—hallucinations; incoherence; anxiety and depression; phobias; history of suicide attempts; "strange affect"; cognitive dysfunction; high potential for violence; history of hospitalizations
Severe—poor judgment; marked organic deficit; "delusions of guilt and persecutions"; "marked depersonalization and derealization"; high potential for violence and/or suicide; "too disturbed to test"; "flat affect"; "very confused and out of touch with reality"; diagnosis of schizophrenia
Source: Unpublished data from interviewer records of screening by Health Services System Office of Mental Health and New York City Human Resources Administration, May 1980.

gleaned from the fact that over half of those so classified were thought to be eligible for SSI (Supplemental Security Income). In only two cases was mental retardation a significant factor.

Discussing the Data

This is, admittedly, a limited data base. It is impossible to gauge the degree of diagnostic precision typical of such a screening effort, nor can this population be taken as representative of homeless men as a whole. Impressionistic evidence, gathered on the street at that time, suggests that among clients of the Men's Shelter, the Wards Island facility was known as a haven for "psychos." Certainly, its isolation and the fact that men are permitted to remain there during the day (a practice not followed in the other public shelters), make it likely that, once there, the more disabled client would find little impetus to leave.

Nonetheless, it is disarming, to say the least, to read the following remarks of Dr. Stanley Hoffman, Director of Research and Evaluation for the New York City Regional Office of Mental Health. Asked to account for the explosive increase in the numbers of homeless men in recent years, he cited the presence — not of expatients — but of "relatively well-educated, relatively well-functioning, well-traveled, middle-class dropouts, who have learned to maneuver the system and who move around" (*New York Times,* June 28, 1981). In this view, he is joined by the Regional Director of the same office, who attributed the increase to "a new generation of urban nomads" (*New York Times,* June 28, 1981). Facile observations such as these fail to distinguish between tramping that is, even today, "practiced out of necessity by the very poor of all ages and [that practiced] out of preference by alienated youth of the privileged classes" (Kett, 1977, p. 272).

More to the point, in light of the findings of the survey summarized above, one may be moved to wonder whether or not the authors of such remarks have ever visited the sites whose residents they describe. Or whether they are familiar with the decision of their own office to deploy on-site mental health teams in all of the public shelters shortly after the survey findings were released. During their first sixteen days, such teams examined 219 men, and — according to Dr. Hoffman himself, curiously enough — found that 25 percent of them were so disturbed as to require immediate hospitalization (New York State Office of Mental Health, April 1981).

Field research conducted over the course of a year (Baxter and Hopper, 1981) lends considerable support to the position that among the secular causes contributing to the rise in the homeless population in the last decade, deinstitutionalization figures prominently. On any number of occasions, young men and women were encountered who either would be counted among those discharged from mental health facilities, or who would be included among the estimated 8,000 a year who were denied entry to such facilities under the tightened admitting criteria in effect since 1968 (New York City Office of the Comptroller, 1979). The following cases, excerpted from field notes, are illustrative:

Penn Station: Long talk with Ed, a young man of 23, with grizzled beard and sunglasses. Quite disturbed—at times tearful—about his situation. Among the snatches I caught, the following: ". . . the Lamb of God, because God wants it that way. It was so much better when I had my apartment: would listen to the radio, have a Marlboro, cup of coffee . . . I always knew I would be someone special, but I never expected this."

We talked in a windswept stairwell, Ed resisting my repeated suggestion to move somewhere warmer. Wolfed down a bagel and a carton of milk, but refused coffee because it made him jittery, speedy. Rapid shifts in conversation and mood: "Do you believe in war?" he asked. To my negative answer, he turns away, then shouts "Armageddon!" and goes on to mumble something about his arm. Slept last night in a warehouse, but can always, when really hard up, return to father's house in Brooklyn for food and clothing. Plagued by the sacrificial image of himself. (3/12/80)

Men's Shelter: Emmet is back on the street again. He had been hospitalized a few months back, but was released some time in late May (at least that's what he told the psychiatrist here). He had been living in a Single Room Occupancy (SRO) uptown, but left after his SSI check failed to arrive on time. Couldn't get it together to go to the welfare office and see what the trouble was. Apparently, no one is following his case outside the hospital. He was told by the clerk here that he was barred from all the hotels because of his record of bad behavior in the past; can't go to Keener Building either because at some point he tangled with a guard there. In effect, he has nowhere to go but the streets. (7/15/80)

Men's Shelter: Often see a young man, Alvin, rummaging through the garbage lining the street in front of the Shelter. One of the "psychos" the staff has no idea of what to do about. All agree he should be hospitalized. None of the hotels will accept him. He won't go to the Keener Building. Sleeps in the doorway until they chase him out, only to come back later. Or catches brief naps on the bathroom floor. Sometimes eats at the Shelter, but mostly subsists on what he finds in the garbage. Tonight, a guard interrupted a conversation I was having with the Shelter's supervisor to report that he had found Alvin "eating the flush out of the toilet." (2/26/80)

Men's Shelter: With one staff member, met and talked with Phillip, a 25-year-old man here since May 1977, at which time according to his records, he was being treated with Thorazine at a clinic in Brooklyn "to relieve nervous tensions." Plans at that time to help him find his own residence apparently fell through. At some point—he isn't clear on this, nor is his record—he was hospitalized. Says he came here from the hospital. A slight, obviously "distracted" young man. Jittery, having some difficulty talking. Appears to be well acquainted with Mental Status exams. When we asked the standard questions (who is the president, what is the date, etc.), he first says he doesn't know, pauses, then—if you wait for it—blurts out the correct answer. Spends his days "just hanging around," sleeps either in the hotels or on the streets, eats in the Shelter. When asked if he in fact sees a social worker once a month, he says "yes," then adds, "See?" and dropping his pants he examines his genitals. Joe (the staff member) gently advises him to pull up his trousers, he does so and skips off to play a round of hopscotch by himself. (7/30/80)

Horace Greeley Square: *Laura said she used to live in a hotel nearby. Apparently ran into lots of varied problems there. Complained of residents who were "really harrassers," elevator doors "with the habit of closing on people," and assorted, if mysterious, assaults on her person. "That hotel has a spirit of its own, if you know what I mean"—and it was clear she felt it to be a menacing one. (7/16/80)*

What is most disheartening in this sorry litany is the realization that the wretched fate accorded many such casualties of bureaucratic bungling and ill-planned fiscal restraint is by no means an inevitable one. This is not to deny the difficulties such individuals present to clinicians charged with their care — by default if not by cruel design. It is rather to lament the shortsightedness, charitably put, of policies that in effect segregate responsibility for essential life supports from responsibility for therapeutic attention. The latest Five-Year Plan of the Mental Health Office (1981), for example, is content simply to assert that "the basic needs of the 'street people'—food, shelter, bath, clothing, medical care—are the responsibility of the social welfare system" (Office of Mental Health, 1981, p. 49). But human needs do not admit of such neat divisions. Here if anywhere, Wing and Olsen's insistence (1979, p. 172) that "there is always an interaction between clinical and social problems [and that] it is rarely possible to separate the two in any way that would be convenient for the development of independent medical and social services" would appear to apply with particular force.

With this in mind, the Office of Mental Health's claim to have "moved aggressively to respond to the mental health needs of people in New York City who are both mentally disabled and homeless" (New York State Office of Mental Health, 1981) can be seen for the acutely limited action it is. The State has put Community Support Service (CSS) teams in the public shelters, deployed a mobile outreach unit, set aside funding for an assessment center, and lent an old hospital building to the city for use as a shelter. But what exactly do such activities amount to? In two years of operation, the CSS team in the men's shelter has managed to place fifteen men in residences off the Bowery; the stigmatizing effects of using erstwhile psychiatric hospitals as shelters should be apparent; and, without appropriate residential backup, outreach and assessment efforts look more and more like the antic displacement activities of animals under stress. What is accomplished when someone is persuaded to come in out of the cold only to learn that there is no room at the inn? The most successful program of outreach to the disabled homeless in New York City repeatedly has attested to the damage done by false promises. Lack of housing and snarls in public assistance, they report, "can jeopardize both the willingness and the ability of many clients to pursue further referrals" (Office of Mental Health, n.d., p. 23). Only the professionally contrary will continue to insist that basic life supports are not, strictly speaking, within the province of "mental health needs."

Even acknowledging the truth of Wing and Olsen's proposition, the difficulties in practicing it are formidable. The situation of labor entry aged men and women who are disabled and dependent is not eased by the opprobrium attached to not working in a job oriented society (Maurer, 1979). With unemployment rates among minority youths in urban areas running as high as 50 percent, the prospects for gainful work in such a population are bleak. Sheltered workshops have their own shortcomings — not least of which is the shame felt by many expatients who are assigned to menial tasks alongside the mentally retarded (Estroff, 1981). Lack of work, meaningful or otherwise, has extended the limbo period of adolescence for thousands of young adults. When combined with recurrent periods of disability or institutionalization, it guarantees a delegitimized existence in the eyes of society. Nor, it is safe to say, have the possible benefits of various forms of "useful unemployment" (Illich, 1977) begun to broach the imagination of program planners.

Before all else, however, the question of appropriate residence must be addressed. As one of our informants puts it: "The most important thing in every man's life is shelter. Once you have shelter, then you are able to get yourself together, then you are able to develop the idea of how you can get yourself out of the trouble you are in" (Isaac, Keener Building, August 1980). This is so obvious an observation that one is hard-pressed to account for the refusal of mental health officials to take seriously their own responsibility in this regard. Without decent, safe, accessible shelter, therapeutic efforts are doomed. What the homeless poor who are mentally disabled need is (1) hospice, a place of refuge, where they can begin to acquire the trust and relearn the skills necessary for sharing household tasks; and (2) supportive residence, where that trust and those skills can be nurtured. These are the basics, without which all talk about outreach, assessment, and reaffiliation is so much smoke.

References

Advisory Social Service Committee of the Municipal Lodging House. *The Men We Lodge.* New York: Advisory Social Service Committee of the Municipal Lodging House, 1915.
Anderson, N. *The Hobo: The Sociology of the Homeless Man.* Chicago: University of Chicago Press, 1923.
Bahr, H. M. (Ed.). *Disaffiliated Man: Essays and Bibliography on Skid Row, Vagrancy, and Outsiders.* Toronto: University of Toronto Press, 1970.
Bahr, H. M. *Skid Row: An Introduction to Disaffiliation.* New York: Oxford University Press, 1973.
Baxter, E., and Hopper, K. "Pathologies of Place and Disorders of Mind." *Health/PAC Bulletin,* 1980, *11* (4), 1-2, 6-12, 21-22.
Baxter, E., and Hopper, K. "The New Mendicancy — Homeless in New York City." September 1981 (submitted for publication).

Bendiner, E. *The Bowery Man.* New York: Thomas Nelson and Sons, 1961.

Caton, C. L. "The New Chronic Patient and the System of Community Care." *Hospital and Community Psychiatry,* 1981, *32* (7), 475–478.

Chafetz, L., and Terry, R. A. "Homelessness and Transiency Among the Chronic Mentally Ill." Paper delivered at the Annual Meeting of the American Orthopsychiatric Association, March 30, 1981.

Estroff, S. *Making It Crazy: An Ethnography of Psychiatric Clients in an American Community.* Berkeley: University of California, 1981.

Haveliwala, Y. "Community Help for the Homeless." *New York Times,* Letter to the Editor, October 8, 1981.

Illich, I. *Toward a History of Needs.* New York: Pantheon, 1977.

Kett, J. E. *Rites of Passage: Adolescence in America 1790 to the Present.* New York: Basic Books, 1977.

Kromer, T. *Waiting for Nothing.* New York: Alfred A. Knopf, 1935.

Manhattan Bowery Corporation. "Shopping Bag Ladies: Homeless Women." New York: Manhattan Bowery Corporation, April 1, 1979.

Maurer, H. *Not Working.* New York: Holt, Rinehart and Winston, 1979.

New York City Office of the Comptroller. *Performance Analysis of Programs of New York State Assistance to New York City Agencies Serving Deinstitutionalized Psychiatric Patients.* New York: New York City Office of the Comptroller, 1979.

New York State Office of Mental Health. *Five Year Comprehensive Plan for Services to the Mentally Ill Persons in New York State.* Albany: New York State Office of Mental Health, 1981.

New York State Office of Mental Health. *Goddard-Riverside Project Reach Out Evaluation Studies.* Albany: New York State Office of Mental Health, n.d.

New York State Office of Mental Health. Internal Memo. Albany, N.Y.: October 12, 1979.

New York State Office of Mental Health. Internal Memo, "Level of Care Distribution of Resident Patients in State Psychiatric Center Adult Units." Albany, N.Y., March 31, 1980.

New York State Office of Mental Health. "Who Are the Homeless Mentally Ill?" *This Month in Mental Health,* April 1981, p. 5.

Pepper, B., Kirshner, M., and Ryglewicz, H. "The Young Adult Chronic Patient: Overview of a Population." *Hospital and Community Psychiatry,* 1981, *32* (7), 463–469.

Polak, P. R., and Kirby, M. W. "A Model to Replace Psychiatric Hospitals." *The Journal of Nervous and Mental Disease,* 1976, *162* (1), 13–22.

Reich, R. "Care of the Chronically Mentally Ill: A National Disgrace." *American Journal of Psychiatry,* 1973, *130,* 911–912.

Reich, R., and Siegel, L. "The Emergence of the Bowery as a Psychiatric Dumping Ground." *Psychiatric Quarterly,* 1978, *50* (3), 191–201.

Rubin, M. "Reducing Disincentives and Fostering the Rehabilitation Process: An Existing Model Program." In L. G. Perlman (Ed.), *Rehabilitation of the Mentally Ill in the 1980s.* Washington, D.C.: National Rehabilitation Association, 1980.

Schwartz, S. R., and Goldfinger, S. M. "The New Chronic Patient: Clinical Characteristics of an Emerging Subgroup." *Hospital and Community Psychiatry,* 1981, *32* (7), 470–474.

Scull, A. *Decarceration: Community Treatment of the Deviant—A Radical View.* Englewood Cliffs, N.J.: Prentice-Hall, 1977.

Segal, S. P., and Baumohl, J. "Engaging the Disengaged: Proposals on Madness and Vagrancy." *Social Work,* 1980, *25* (5), 358–365.

Segal, S. P., Baumohl, J., and Johnson, E. "Falling Through the Cracks: Mental Disorder and Social Margin in a Young Vagrant Population." *Social Problems,* 1977, *24* (3), 387–400.

42

Talbott, J. A. "Care of the Chronically Mentally Ill—Still a National Disgrace." *American Journal of Psychiatry,* 1979, *136,* 688–689.

Test, M. A., and Stein, L. I. "Practical Guidelines for the Community Treatment of Markedly Impaired Patients." *Community Mental Health Journal,* 1976, *12* (1), 42–82.

Wallace, S. E. *Skid Row as a Way of Life.* Totowa, N.J.: Bedminster Press, 1965.

Wing, J. K., and Olsen, R. "Principles of the New Community Care." In J. K. Wing and R. Olsen (Eds.), *Community Care for the Mentally Disabled.* New York: Oxford University Press, 1979.

Kim Hopper, Ellen Baxter, and Stuart Cox are researchers at Community Service Society in New York City and members of the Coalition for the Homeless.

Chronic disability is not an inevitable consequence of chronic mental disorders. The risk of developing chronic disability is dependent upon the response of the psychosocial environment, including the pattern of clinical care.

Social Breakdown in Young Adults: Keeping Crises from Becoming Chronic

Ernest M. Gruenberg

We are seeing new cases of chronic disability among people who have never been patients in a chronic institution or even in any hospital. Chronic disability is not an inevitable consequence of chronic mental disorders. The changed mental life and the associated disabilities are not mechanically linked. The disabilities are in psychosocial life; their manifestations are the same in many disorders. These disabilities are decreases in abilities which are learned in the course of socialization into the human community.

Chronic disability continues to occur even without chronic institutionalization. The deinstitutionalization enthusiasts sometimes seem to believe that if people with chronic mental disorders avoid chronic institutional placement in mental hospitals they will never show chronic disability. This chapter will present new cases which show this to be a false assumption for which there has never been any evidence. The available evidence shows that, if the psychiatric service system responds to an episode of decompensation in personal and social functioning with a rapid, relevant response that is designed to preserve the individual's network of social support relationships and community support system relationships, the risk that this episode of decompensation will become chronic is greatly reduced (Gruenberg, 1969, 1974).

B. Pepper, H. Ryglewicz (Eds.). *New Directions for Mental Health Services: The Young Adult Chronic Patient,* no. 14. San Francisco: Jossey-Bass, June 1982.

Many now recognize that the deinstitutionalization enthusiasm, which has resulted in a wide scattering of mental health center services, avoidance of chronic mental hospital care, and crisis intervention operations, has not succeeded in rehabilitating all of those who were formerly chronically disabled. It has also failed to prevent the development of new cases of chronic disability among mentally disordered individuals. These new cases of chronically disabled individuals are predominantly among young people who have developed their adult roles in a period when chronic institutionalization has not been available. These cases demonstrate more than anything else the fact that our current technology is inadequate for the total prevention of cases of chronic disability among those with chronic mental disorders.

The studies by Bert Pepper in Rockland County, New York (see Chapter One, this volume) have shown beyond a doubt that these young people are a growing and important group of chronically disabled patients. There are a number of reasons why this group of new chronic mental patients has first become clearly visible in Rockland County. I wish to mention two of them. First, Rockland County was one of the very first American counties to set up a comprehensive community mental health program within its county government. That was twenty-five years ago, very shortly after the passage of the New York State 1954 Community Mental Health Services Act. Second, Rockland County is fortunate to have Pepper as the Commissioner in that he has long been alert to the problem of the chronically disabled patient and thinks not only in clinical terms but in community-wide and community service organizational terms.

Chronic Disability Versus Chronic Disorder

Chronic disability and chronic mental disorder are not synonymous. The term *chronic* is properly applied to conditions which last a long time. Many mental disorders do not lead to significant disability. These are often referred to as *minor*. Certain kinds of nondisabling phobias, panic disorders, dysthymia, and obsessions do not lead to significant losses of function. That is not to say that they do not cause distress and are not suitable targets for treatment. Such conditions can interfere with optimal development without producing actual disabilities. Sigmund Freud (1937) once wrote a paper entitled "Analysis, Terminable and Interminable," describing cases with anxiety and tension who were not only self-supporting, self-caring, and not causing significant trouble to others, they were actually supporting the analyst. The problem was simply in terminating the relationship with the analyst.

But it is not only minor disorders that do not lead to significant disability. There are people with schizophreniform disorders who may be somewhat limited in achieving their maximum potential and have the residual symptoms of short temper, irritability, sleep disturbance, and so on, who are not significantly disabled in their personal and social functioning. People with manic depressive disorders have acute episodes of mood disorder but in the long term are not disabled; many are unusually productive, creative, and highly able people.

We do know, however, that people with chronic mental disorders are at an increased risk of developing chronic disability, and systematic studies have shown that the size of this risk is dependent upon the response of the psychosocial environment, including the pattern of clinical care, to the presence of the underlying disorder. The early studies with which I was associated showed that what was called the social breakdown syndrome is not as likely to become chronic if the response is good community care. Community care means that the response to acute episodes of the social breakdown syndrome is carefully organized to reduce the period of inpatient care and to preserve the individual's link to the community support system and the intimate social support system. The social breakdown syndrome was defined as a form of disability in which work functions, self-care functions or recreation functions fell to a totally inadequate level, or in which intolerable, aggressive, destructive behavior developed. These episodes of social breakdown syndrome are mostly acute and short-lived but some become chronic, and, as was stated, this proportion is dependent upon the pattern of care (Gruenberg, 1969, 1974).

The deinstitutionalization movement leaders have tended to act and think as though the prevention of chronic institutionalization would prevent all cases of the chronic social breakdown syndrome. This is contrary to the empirical evidence on such matters. What we do know is that optimal community care which minimizes the disruption of the individual's links to family and community will prevent about two thirds of the cases. But the best programs cannot prevent the other third of the new cases of chronic social breakdown syndrome from occurring.

This reflects the weakness of our current technology. Undoubtedly, some of the new cases of chronic disability which are arising among people with mental disorders today are due to a failure to apply the best treatment techniques available at the time of acute episodes. However, in the presence of good programs, in general, the bulk of the new cases probably reflect, in my judgment, the inadequacy of our present treatment techniques.

Figure 1 shows that in an adult population of 100,000 people (aged sixteen to sixty-five) one can expect annually some 500 or 600 episodes of acute social breakdown syndrome. The curve shows that the episodes usually last one to six weeks and that by the time three months have passed the bulk of them have recovered. What one can see is that the cases which became chronic numbered about forty-six before the reform in the organization of psychiatric services and the development of community care programs. In those episodes which began after two years of the community care program, less than sixteen per year became chronic, that is, lasted more than one year.

This is the nature of the improved experience which community care programs can be expected to produce with modern techniques of ·treatment

Figure 1. Episodes of Social Breakdown Syndrome

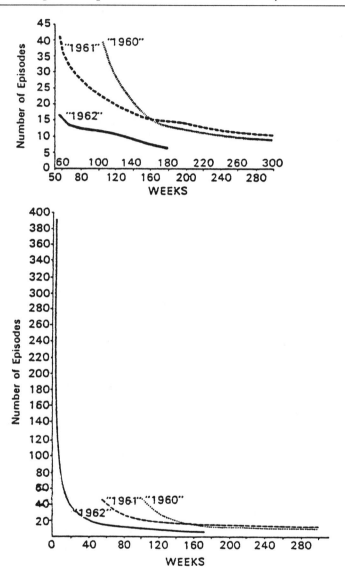

Estimated number of episodes of social breakdown syndrome lasting more than the specified number of weeks arising in the population of Dutchess County (ages 16 to 65) during "1960," "1961," and "1962." The *top section* is the vertical scale amplified four times.

Source: Gruenberg, E. M., Snow, H. B., and Bennett, C. L. "Preventing the Social Breakdown Syndrome." In F. C. Redlich (Ed.), *Social Psychiatry.* Baltimore: Williams and Wilkens, 1969.

and good community based services. The sixteen chronic cases (lasting more than one year) which develop each year have a very poor prognosis. They do not tend to recover. Good rehabilitation programs, though, make some difference. But we do not have any reason to think that a substantial proportion will begin to function adequately in self-care, work, or recreation activities without causing various troubles to those around them. It is on this group that we must focus our attention in the immediate future.

The Nature of the Disabilities

Disabilities, handicaps, and impairments have been described throughout the history of health services and health research. But unlike the diagnoses of disorders, there has never been any attempt at a standard nomenclature with respect to them. In 1980 the World Health Organization (WHO) issued a supplement to the International Classification of Diseases offering a standardized definition of these terms (WHO, 1980). Unfortunately, the WHO usage is at some variance with common American uses of these terms, but the concepts to which they refer are largely in harmony with American usage. I offer here a brief summary of the WHO classification for the purposes of this chapter and for clarification of the later discussion of the disabilities we see in these chronically disabled young patients.

Impairment is a defect in the function or presence of an organ. In physical medicine it can apply to a paralyzed limb or an amputated limb or to blindness or deafness. In mental functioning, it applies to brain and personality functions in their most isolated form. That is, there can be an impaired ability to recall earlier experiences, to process information, to grasp a new idea, to integrate conflicting signals from the environment, to control impulses toward disorganized or violent behavior, to solve IQ type problems, and so on. These are examples of impairment.

Disability refers to activities. We are familiar with the concept derived from physical rehabilitation of the activities of daily living often abbreviated as ADL. This refers to the self-care of getting dressed in an appropriate fashion, toileting, eating, keeping one's body clean, and so forth. This is in contrast to soiling, being disheveled, unkempt, undressed, self-neglectful, and so on. Disabilities also occur in work functions. These include employment but also other kinds of work. In a statement being prepared for the American Medical Association by the American Psychiatric Association, work is referred to as anything needed by the social group which, if that individual does not do it, somebody else will do it. This includes housekeeping, child care, care of the ill and disabled, household maintenance, yard work, and so on.

This broadened idea of work beyond employment is very important in order to be clear about the nature of work disability. It is important for two reasons. First, it is important to recognize that many people do work outside of employment. It is socially useful work which must be evaluated in addition to employability. If anyone is to do research on the frequency of disability, their index for research must be independent of the local unemployment rate. Second, many people undertake their major work roles outside the employment market. This is particularly true of women who devote themselves to maintaining households and rearing children.

But men and women do not live by bread alone. What makes life worth living is not simply the matter of self-care and contributing to socially useful work. The really important things in life have to do with recreation, festivities, and other embroideries of our lives which some people call play. These important activities include reading, writing, taking part in parties, entertaining of others, participation in worship and other church functions, the playing of cards, dancing, and so on. The ability to enjoy is an important ability. Some people who are chronically disabled have lost their ability to enjoy life and shared social interactions with other people.

In summary, there are four areas of disability: self-care, work, recreation, and control of socially unacceptable troublesome impulses.

Handicap as used by WHO refers to a loss of opportunity to participate in the social organization of the previously-noted activities. Handicap arises at the interface between the disabled person and the society's physical and social environment. A blind person who has learned to use a seeing eye dog and a cane but is not acceptable to employers as a telephone operator or stenographer is handicapped. A former mental hospital patient who is not acceptable to a school, club, or an employer because of the history of having been in a mental hospital is handicapped. Handicaps are socially imposed barriers to participation in the community's life on the basis of the person's impairment or disability. We are sensitive to the fact that these barriers are modifiable and, in fact, should be modified. Mainstreaming is an effort to end a period of handicap in social role participation among people with developmental disabilities. In extreme situations, handicap can occur in the absence of any impairment, disability, or disease. The untouchables of India and the child in the black slum have handicaps totally unrelated to their abilities.

Therefore, handicaps can be reduced by changes in social practices. Disabilities can be reduced by compensatory mechanisms which the individual can develop or can be helped to develop through retraining. Impairments can be reduced through a variety of prosthetic devices. The lame can use canes and crutches and artificial limbs. The person whose anxiety interferes with problem-solving can have the anxiety reduced through the use of medication and thereby be able to come into more realistic relationships with the issues of their daily life. The cognitively impaired can use paper and pencil to make lists of things the rest of us find easy to remember, and can have calendars at many locations to remind them of the date and clocks at many locations to remind them of the time. Cognitively impaired individuals who have trouble remembering where things are at night can leave the light on to help them in their orientation to the physical world. Those are the types of prostheses available to reduce the impact of the impairment. Whenever impairment is reduced, disability is reduced to some extent. Reducing disability helps to reduce handicap.

The disabilities which have been discussed in this chapter are disabilities in the WHO sense. We are referring here to losses of ability. Keeping oneself clean, dressed, and presentable and feeding oneself is necessary. These abilities are not present in the newborn. They are acquired skills. Work is also an acquired skill. Some mental disorders lead to a loss in these skills or abilities. The ability to play is present in very small infants in some sense. But most of the recreational activities which we value most highly are also socially learned during the process of maturation and socialization. They do not develop automatically with the development of the higher central nervous system but are part of the social heritage which each person acquires within the context of their own personality development and individuation. It is important to recognize that these abilities which are lost when disability arises are socially acquired skills. It is probably for that reason that they are so sensitive to disruptions in the social context in which the individual is living. Some of these abilities tend to deteriorate when the social network is interrupted. This would suggest that they are not only acquired through the process of socialization but maintained through the continuity of social and interpersonal relationships.

It is necessary in the individual case to make a distinction between the loss of the socially acquired abilities and the failure to develop them. Some of the young, new, chronically disabled people have had mental disorders which have more or less led to a loss of these abilities. But others have never acquired certain vital abilities. They have never learned to work, or they have never learned to care for themselves, or they have never learned to take part in organized recreation, or they have failed to develop the necessary control of violent and troublesome impulses. It is important to distinguish these two groups of chronically disabled individuals because the treatment programs will be significantly different. In general, the outlook is better for people who have lost the abilities and have a basis for relearning them or compensating for the impairments which have developed as a consequence of the mental disorder. For those who have never developed these abilities, the whole process of delayed development and socialization must be approached with the notion that it will be a long and slow process and, of course, dependent upon the original reason why these abilities have not been previously developed.

This whole discussion is simply an attempt to sort out the issues associated with the new chronically disabled individual in the mental health services. It is a growing population for various reasons and points to the inadequacies of our current techniques for helping people with serious mental disorders. We should not lose heart because of these individuals' continued appearance in our service programs. Their numbers are smaller than thirty years ago, which represents an advance. They point our attention to unresolved scientific and tech-

50

nical problems. They also challenge our civilization to decide how best to care for those who have never learned how to care for themselves or have lost the ability to care for themselves. These new chronic mentally disabled individuals are the new challenge to the mental health movement.

References

Freud, S. "Analysis, Terminable and Interminable." In J. Strachey (Ed.), *The Standard Edition of the Complete Works of Sigmund Freud.* Vol. 23. London: Hogarth and the Institute of Psychoanalysis, 1953. (Originally published 1937.)
Gruenberg, E. M. "From Practice to Theory: Community Mental Health Services and the Nature of Psychoses." *Lancet,* April 5, 1969, 721-724.
Gruenberg, E. M. "The Social Breakdown Syndrome and Its Prevention." In G. Caplan (Ed.), *American Handbook of Psychiatry.* Vol. 2: *Child and Adolescent Psychiatry, Sociocultural and Community Psychiatry.* (2nd ed.) New York: Basic Books, 1974.
World Health Organization. *International Classification of Impairments, Disabilities, and Handicaps.* Geneva: World Health Organization, 1980.

Ernest M. Gruenberg is professor, Department of Mental Hygiene, Johns Hopkins School of Hygiene and Public Health and professor of psychiatry, Johns Hopkins University School of Medicine.

The impact of psychotropic medications on the course of illness varies depending on premorbid functioning. The effect on relapse rate of low-dosage maintenance needs to be examined in the hopes of minimizing its side effects.

Psychopharmacology: Special Considerations

Donald F. Klein

A lot of what is going on in our field and in our society with regard to the care of the chronically mentally ill can be understood as the direct impact, during the middle 1950s, of the development of antipsychotic medication, and its effect on our system or various nonsystems of care. I had the fortune to start out as a first year psychiatric resident at Creedmoor State Hospital in 1953 when we didn't have medications. The place was in actuality a well-meaning jail and custodial institution. The psychiatric aspect of it was that electroconvulsive therapy (ECT) and nursing sometimes worked.

Over the next few years, antipsychotics came in. In 1955, I was first exposed to antipsychotics while running a ward of World War I veterans who had been hospitalized for thirty continuous years or more. We were given supplies of a new experimental compound called chlorpromazine and gave them at the time what was considered a high dose of 200 mg/day. One man came over to me after several weeks and said, "Well, Doc, when am I getting out of here?" That was the first time that he had said anything in thirty years. It was literally the most astonishing experience of my psychiatric life, because it is not often that you see an authentic miracle. That was the initial attitude many had about antipsychotic medication. We first viewed it as a wonder drug which would do miraculous things.

In fact, these drugs do miraculous things. But, as we have learned in

B. Pepper, H. Ryglewicz (Eds.). *New Directions for Mental Health Services: The Young Adult Chronic Patient,* no. 14. San Francisco: Jossey-Bass, June 1982.

the past twenty-five years, they are not for everybody, not all the time, and not under all circumstances.

It is important that antipsychotic medication be seen against the background of what we know from the nineteenth century with regard to mental illness. It was obvious back in Kraepelin's day that schizophrenia was essentially a deteriorative disease. Recovery was rare and occurred probably in no more than 8 to 10 percent of the patients in Kraepelin's day. Complete recovery was (and is) a reconstitution with no social, psychological, or cognitive deficits. A second kind of recovery was continued symptomatic complaints with considerable social and cognitive deficit, but not so much that the person could not be out of the hospital. The third type of outcome was the patient who had made a very incomplete or no recovery, had a very marked deficit with continuing symptomatology and had to be kept in the hospital.

What happens to these three categories of patients with the advent of medication? Our hope, the hope of all of us, is that the first category would increase radically, and that we would be able to create more people who came to complete recovery without deficit. But I think the consensus of the experts is that the actual proportion of people who recover without deficit probably has not increased since Kraepelin's day. What has actually happened is that the number of patients in the second category has increased enormously. It is very much the second category patients who are the subject of our discussions about the young adult chronic patient. Therefore, it is very important that we focus upon medication, in both its positive and negative aspects, as probably responsible both for deinstitutionalization and for the creation of the group of young chronic patients in their present social form. What can we say about these second category patients and their prognosis?

There have been an enormous number of studies with regard to who is going to end up well and who is not. These studies can be summed up quickly: There are two psychoses that are of major importance. The psychosis of manic-depressive disease is characterized by a very marked shift in mood and activation, so that the person may become high as a kite and disorganized, or become depressed, inept, and unable to carry out the performance of day-to-day living. Now, the major thing about manic-depressive disease is that, although the patients can become extremely ill, nonfunctioning, often suicidal or actual suicide cases, their prognosis for recovery from the episode is excellent, and chances of their becoming completely restored to normal and able to pick up their roles in life are also excellent. The role medication plays is a major benefit in shortening the period of illness, but does not really affect the level of functioning between episodes.

What Kraepelin (1971) pointed out was that the other group of psychotic patients, who are now called schizophrenic, are people who have episodes, but even if their psychosis goes away, between episodes there is a marked deficit. Further, with recurrent psychotic episodes the deficit becomes progressively worse. These patients typically do not have motivation; their social and sexual feelings decrease. They don't go out socially, and, if they were previously ambitious, this characteristic becomes badly damaged.

The bottom line of medication benefit is that, the closer the psychotic person is to a manic-depressive, the better off he is once his psychosis has remitted. Therefore, if you must be psychotic, be manic. The patient who has good premorbid development, who has an acute onset of his illness, whose illness is characterized largely by overactivation or very marked retardation — even though he has many of the signs often associated with schizophrenia, such as delusions — will usually respond well to medication.

The antipsychotic medications, like the antidepressants, do not make the patient into a different person; what they do is to shorten the period of florid illness very markedly, and therefore save the patient from enormous pain and trouble.

The issue of premorbidity is important. Typically, the person who becomes depressed, or manic, is a solid citizen; that is, prior to the illness he or she is not far outside of the range of normal functioning.

The more a person deviates from his peers, the worse is the prognosis. The worst form of schizophrenia is schizophrenia characterized by premorbid asociality. If, as a child of five, six, or seven years old, one doesn't get along with other kids in school, is friendless and rejected, and becomes schizophrenic usually in the late teens, one is likely to respond poorly to antipsychotic medication and to go through a life of parasitism and social incompetence despite the use of medication (which usually does, however, block the acute psychotic exacerbations).

These premorbid asocial people are of interest from various points of view. One of the striking things is that they may have a low hereditary loading. We don't have that firmly established yet, but these people seem to stick out in their families like sore thumbs. They are also loaded with neurological soft signs, as noted by Quitkin and Rifkin (1976), in comparison with other schizophrenics. They are also more deviant on neuropsychology tests. A scale of premorbid asociality developed by Gittelman-Klein and Klein (1969) was applied in Washington, D.C., by Wyatt's group (Weinberger and others, 1980), who found that premorbid asociality correlated with ventricular dilation, as measured by the CAT scan. This may imply that this sort of brain damage antecedes the manifest psychosis and is reflected in the peculiar chronic social defect.

Another possibility relevant to the young chronic patient, which has never really been demonstrated, is that the actual experience of being psychotic is in itself brain-damaging. Certainly, the natural history of the illness is that many schizophrenic patients who have one episode go back to work. After another episode, they work partially; and after a third episode it becomes impossible to go back to work. Now that could be demoralization, it could be stigma, it may be exclusion from the work force. All of these social and psychological reasons are possible causes of social incompetence. My own belief from working with such patients for over twenty-five years is that they have brain damage, and that we cannot explain their deterioration in purely socio-psychological terms.

Therefore, the course of brain damage may be extremely important in dealing with these patients. The asocial child may have started out with brain damage, so that his prognosis is difficult to alter. However, we have some hope that, with schizophrenic patients with a good premorbid level of functioning, if we terminate the psychotic episode with medication quickly and effectively, we may shorten the period of active brain injury and thus improve the long-term prognosis. As far as I know, there has never been an adequate clinical trial to test this hypothesis.

Another aspect of the situation is that, for many of the young chronic patients, medication not only has antipsychotic effects, it also has prophylactic effects with regard to psychotic relapse.

Again, Rifkin and Quitkin (Rifkin and others, 1975, 1977) have done several studies in which patients who have been well maintained as outpatients for six months are then either switched to a placebo or maintained on medication. What we have found is that in this outpatient group, over 70 percent relapse within the year on placebo, whereas only 10 percent do so on continued medication.

Perhaps the reason for the high level of relapse in the community is very simply that those who relapse are not taking medication. Therefore, one thing to do is to treat them with long-acting, injectable antipsychotics—patients get one injection every two weeks, and we don't have to worry about their fluctuating level of compliance and cooperation.

One issue of particular importance for young adult patients is whether continued prophylactic medication may be toxic. What are the possibilities, and types of harm, that these medications incur? One type is a condition referred to as *akinesia*. Akinesia is an extrapyramidal side effect of antipsychotic medication. It results in a state of diminished spontaneity. The person is less likely to take action, less likely to pursue goals, and less likely to find rewards.

Unfortunately, that condition is a great deal like the deficit state that occurs in postpsychotic schizophrenia. It is often difficult to tell the two apart on the basis of symptomatology. It is possible, however, to give antiparkinson medication and see if this alleviates the problem. There is little evidence that community patients treated chronically with medication are often suffering from akinesia which would contribute to a nonfunctioning state. In one study we had patients on either placebo or medication. If the medication was an akinetic drag on the patient, then the social functioning of the patient on medication should actually have been inferior to the social functioning of the patient on placebo—at least up to the point when the placebo patients relapsed. But we found that prior to relapse, the placebo-treated patient did just as well as, but not better than, the drug-treated patient. This small amount of data indicates that akinesia may not be a major source of social disability for the drug-maintained patient.

The second kind of side effect, tardive dyskinesia (TD), is a real headache. Tardive dyskinesia is a chronic neurological disorder that occurs in some portion of patients who are usually exposed to antipsychotic medication for a long period of time. This side effect results in chewing, thrusting, and tongue-waggling motions. It does not go away when the medication is stopped unless we detect TD right at the point of onset.

However, in the effort to avoid TD we may take away from the patient the very medication he or she needs to remain sane and functional. The answer to TD will come from research. A new drug, clozapine, which was an effective antipsychotic without extrapyramidal symptoms, was very promising. Unfortunately, agranulocytosis, a severe blood disorder, occurred in patients during its use, and therefore the medication had to be discontinued from clinical trials. We hope that a similar drug will be developed that will not involve such side effects.

One other possibility is to treat the patient with the least amount of medication needed. To find out the minimum medication a patient needs clinically, we progressively lower the dosage and hope to get away with it.

John Kane and his colleagues (1979) at Hillside took a group of patients similar to those he already knew would relapse on placebo. Fifty such patients were put on fluphenazine decanoate at only one-tenth the usual dose. The usual dose is about 25 mg every two weeks, so these patients were getting about 2.5 mg every two weeks. The relapse rate was between the low rate possible with the full dosage of medication and the high rate on placebo. The evidence that even this small dose may be useful for some patients gives us some encouragement.

Another interesting thing was the quality of the relapse between the groups. With the patients placed on placebo, the relapse was abrupt; about half required hospitalization. However, the patients on the very low dose developed a slow roller: Over several weeks they became progressively more peculiar and more socially isolated, said more strange things, and eventually became psychotic. At that point, we were able to raise the medication and put a stop to the psychosis without hospitalization.

These results raise the possibility of a different strategy for the management of chronically ill patients: low-dose medication as their usual form of treatment, with occasional high dosage at the point of relapse. That approach has yet to be tested in an extensive way. Obviously, we all hope that patients getting a very low dose of medication would be less likely to develop TD and other side effects of medication. But we cannot be sure that this is true.

Let me make a more general social statement about the impact of medication on our society and our care of the mentally ill. Our society, with regard to the care of the adult, essentially takes two opposing attitudes: one is that the adult can take care of himself, and that it would be an act of despotism to interfere and to tell him how he should live his life. The other attitude is that this fellow is awfully ill, he is so ill that he is not making any sense and can't take care of himself. Further, he may be a danger to himself or to others. At that point, we commit him in his own best interest, in order to take care of him to the point where he is no longer committable. At that point we are back to the first attitude. So we have essentially two ways of dealing with people: we treat adults either as competent and independent, or as committable. Unfortunately, it turns out that a substantial proportion of the mentally ill, who are treatable with medication, clearly end up in a condition such that they really are taking poor care of themselves, but at the same time are not psychotic. What we have here is a conflict of two social values: respect for autonomy on the one hand, and benevolence on the other.

I have been talking with Bert Pepper about this patient group with various lawyers, phrasing the question, "What do you do about this guy who happens to be recurrently ill but not currently psychotic? He's not taking his medicine, and I know very well that in the next couple of months he will end up re-hospitalized. Is there anything available analogous to the Person In Need of Supervision, a category often used for adolescents?"

No one has liked this idea; I don't like it much myself, but unless there is some constructive approach toward developing some benevolent—if interfering—way that would safeguard such people, they will continue to end up with repeated psychosis and further deterioration. Perhaps repeated hospitalization, despite systematic efforts at aftercare, could be made the legal grounds for such a distasteful abridgement of personal liberty.

References

Gittelman-Klein, R. K., and Klein, D. F. "Premorbid Asocial Adjustment and Prognosis in Schizophrenia." *Journal of Psychiatric Research,* 1969, *7,* 35-53.

Kane, J., and others. "Low-Dose Fluphenazine Decanoate in Maintenance Treatment of Schizophrenics." *Psychiatry Research,* 1979, *1,* 341-348.

Quitkin, F., Rifkin, A., and Klein, D. F. "Neurological Soft Signs in Schizophrenia and Character Disorder (Organicity in Schizophrenia with Premorbid Asociality and Emotionally Unstable Character Disorder)." *Archives of General Psychiatry,* 1976, *33,* 845-853.

Rifkin, A., Quitkin, F., and Klein, D. F. "Akinesia: A Poorly Recognized Drug-Induced Extrapyramidal Behavior Disorder." *Archives of General Psychiatry,* 1975, *32,* 672-674.

Rifkin, A., and others. "Fluphenazine Decanoate, Fluphenazine Hydrochloride Given Orally, and Placebo in Remitted Schizophrenics. I. Relapse Rate After One Year." *Archives of General Psychiatry,* 1977, *34,* 43-47.

Weinberger, D. R., and others. "Poor Premorbid Adjustment and C.A.T. Scan Abnormalities in Chronic Schizophrenics." *American Journal of Psychiatry,* 1980, *137,* 1410-1413.

Wender, P. H., and Klein, D. F. *Mind, Mood, and Medicine: A Guide to the New Biopsychiatry.* New York: Farrar, Straus, and Giroux, 1981.

Donald F. Klein is director of psychiatric research at New York State Psychiatric Institute and professor of psychiatry at the College of Physicians and Surgeons, Columbia University.

Programs serving the chronically mentally ill in Dane County,
Wisconsin involve assertive outreach to the patient
and the community.

Community Treatment of the Young Adult Patient

Leonard I. Stein
Mary Ann Test

We are in the midst of a revolution in mental health care for the chronic mentally ill person; that revolution has been called the deinstitutionalization movement. The major beneficiaries of the deinstitutionalization movement are not
the people who have been deinstitutionalized; instead, the major beneficiaries
will be the future generations of persons who will be suffering from severe and
chronic mental illness. The present young adult chronic patient is the first post-
deinstitutionalized generation of persons suffering from severe chronic mental
illness, and it is with this population that we will be setting the stage for how
people with chronic mental illness will live from now on. We are, in fact,
changing the system; will the result be much as the deinstitutionalized population are now living—living on the streets out of a bag; living in a single room
occupancy; living in board-and-care homes, staring at television sets—or can
it be better than that (Allen, 1976; Lamb and Goertzel, 1971)? Our experience
in Dane County, Wisconsin, would indicate that it indeed can be better (Stein
and Test, 1980). This chapter reports some of what we are doing in Dane
County. It is not being presented as a model to be precisely duplicated, but instead to explicate principles and guidelines that can be used to shape the services that best fit your situation and needs.

    Dane County has a population of about 300,000 people and has identi-

B. Pepper, H. Ryglewicz (Eds.). *New Directions for Mental Health Services: The Young Adult*
Chronic Patient, no. 14. San Francisco: Jossey-Bass, June 1982.

fied a thousand people suffering from chronic mental illness. Approximately 40 percent of those are between the ages of thirteen and thirty-five; thus we have a significant number of young chronic mentally ill people. A sizable percentage of those have not seen the inside of a state hospital, and a number have not been hospitalized at all. Nevertheless, they suffer from the significant disabilities inherent in chronic mental illness. The relatively small amount of hospital time in their medical histories is due to the fact that they are younger and have come into the system since we have been involved in developing alternatives to mental hospital programs.

Community Programs

We have learned that working with this difficult population requires a programmatic approach. We have a variety of programs which will be briefly described. This allows us to reserve most of the chapter to elaborate the principles and the guidelines that we use in working with patients and the community to help this group of people make a stable adjustment to community life.

We have a very active crisis intervention unit that is mobile, staffed twenty-four hours a day, seven days a week, and indeed does crisis resolution, not just triage. In addition, we have a mobile community treatment team (MCT) that specializes in working with the more difficult to treat chronic patient. Almost all of their patients fall within the eighteen to thirty-five age group. This is a team that operates seven days a week, two shifts a day, with the crisis intervention unit taking over for the midnight to 8:00 A.M. shift. We have a day treatment program, cooperative apartments, medication clinics, support groups, and an out-patient therapy clinic. Thus we have a cluster of programs that work cooperatively in managing this patient group.

Patient Disabilities

Prior to describing our intervention strategies, we will summarize the disabilities and needs the patients have and how the disabilities interfere with their getting those needs fulfilled. The disabilities that we find in our patients are as follows:
1. High vulnerability to stress;
2. Extreme dependency;
3. Deficiency in coping skills;
4. Difficulty with interpersonal relationships;
5. Concrete thinking/anxiety in new situations: Both of these disabilities impair patients' ability to generalize learning; that is, what they learn in one setting is difficult to put into practice in another setting.
These disabilities interfere with patients' attempts to organize and maintain those needs that are necessary to establish a stable adjustment to

community life. The needs are quite obvious; in essence they need exactly what the rest of us do (Turner and Shifren, 1979). They need a place to live; they need an opportunity to socialize; they need some kind of meaningful vocational or avocational activity that anchors their day, gives them a reason to get up in the morning, and gives some meaning to their lives; they need finances; medical services; mental health services and crisis intervention services. Their only need that the rest of us do not specifically require is support directed at the community in which they live. The community must be helped to learn how to accept their presence and accept them as members. Any treatment organization that works with this population must understand that supporting the community is just as important as providing support to patients.

Principles and Guidelines of Community Treatment

The following section will outline guidelines and principles that we use in working with this patient population. However, first we would like to give you an overriding and fundamental principle: the primary locus of care must be in the community. That does not mean that the hospital is not one important element in the total number of services that are needed by this population. It simply means, for example, that when the patient is hospitalized, the community team follows the patient into the hospital and shares responsibility for developing the hospital treatment plan with the hospital staff. And, it is the community team that makes the discharge plan and determines when the patient should be discharged.

Working with the Patient

An Assertive Approach. Frequently patients do not seem to be motivated to stay involved with the treatment program. In fact, what is most frustrating about their willingness to be involved is that it is highly variable. There are times when a patient will seek help; at other times the same patient does not want to have anything to do with you or your medication. To accept being fired by the patient with a shrug of the shoulders and a comment that "unmotivated people can't be helped" is, in essence, evidence of poor clinical judgment. Lack of motivation or variability in motivation is part of the basic illness. If this lack is passively accepted, that person, within a relatively short period of time and in all probability, will again regress into a psychosis, be hospitalized, and be referred back to start all over again.

Our programs are assertive in keeping patients involved. If someone does not show up for an appointment or for his job (we have a very careful monitoring system to keep us apprised of that), we will go out and find the person. We may have to go to his home; we may have to drive along the street we know he frequents. When we find the client, we don't hit him (or her) over the head, shanghai him, and haul him back into the program; but we do stop him, talk to him, and try to convince him that we would really like to get reinvolved with him. The patient may say no the first few times we try, but in our experience he will eventually come back into the program. This approach has markedly reduced dropouts from our programs.

Individually Tailored Programming. Patients have a wide variety of needs. To help provide these needs in the most efficient way possible, we operate by individualizing programming. We do not give everybody everything. Because we have only so much energy, time, and resources, we thereby meet the needs of each individual patient, and at the same time make the most efficient use of our resources.

In-Vivo Services. We noted earlier that many of our patients do not transfer learning from one place to another very well. Let us give you some concrete examples. We used to teach patients how to cook in the model kitchen in the hospital and to shop in the supermarket near the hospital. After discharge, we visited patients and found they were not shopping in their local supermarkets or using the stoves in their kitchens. We tried to find out why, and learned that when they went to their local supermarket they found that the aisles were labeled A, B, C, D, and E, instead of 1, 2, 3, and 4. In addition, they said, they tried finding what they wanted but the products were not in the aisles that they expected to find them in; they next noticed that people were staring at them. Needless to say, they left the supermarket as fast as they could and did not go back.

The reasons for not using their stove, even if they had found food, were similar. In the hospital's kitchen there are beautiful modern stoves, unlike those in their poverty-level apartments. Again, they could not transfer their learning.

We learned from these experiences to carefully assess patients' skills, to determine which ones might be generalized, and to teach these in a group setting. But for those patients who were not able to generalize this knowledge, we had to go to their homes and neighborhoods to teach them how to cook in their kitchens, to shop in their supermarkets, to use the specific bus routes they needed to get from home to their sheltered workshop placement, and so on.

Capitalizing on Patients' Strength. We learned that we got much better results if we paid attention to patients' strengths instead of spending all of our time on their pathology. For an example, Mary got a job as a maid in a motel. One of our workers spent two or three days working side by side with her and helping her learn how to do the various tasks that she had to do. Then he weaned himself away from her and things went well for one day; on the second day we received a phone call. The patient said, "I have got to get back to the hospital." We said, "What's the matter, Mary?" She said, "The T.V. set in every room I walk into is controlling my mind and telling me what to do." That particular delusion is a common one for Mary to develop during a psychosis. Rather than ask her about how her delusions related to her early life experiences, we asked her, what happened today? She replied that nothing had happened. We told her that she was obviously upset about something, and asked again what happened. She finally told us that the supervisor said she doesn't know how to make the beds correctly. We told her that we would be right over. One of our mental health aides went down and checked with the supervisor and, sure enough, Mary wasn't making the corners on the bed the way the supervisor wanted them made. The aide spent another day with Mary helping her learn how to better make the corners on the bed. After she learned that and was complimented by the supervisor, the voices from the television set stopped telling her what to do. We continue to find that it is useful to focus on the strengths of our patients rather than spending too much time on pathology.

Titered Support. Over and over again we have heard that it is harmful to allow patients to get overdependent. Although that is certainly true, the fact is that they are dependent and require support. Most of them are going to be dependent on us for the rest of their lives to a greater or lesser degree. The strategy is to increase the independence to the greatest degree possible but not beyond what the patient can tolerate. To do this requires good clinical judgment. The amount of support given is highly variable and is dependent on the patient's current clinical need. For example, there will be some days we will give a person a great deal more support than we will two days later or two weeks later. In summary, the patient needs support, and good clinical judgment must be utilized in order to titer the support so that patients get what they need but not more.

Relating to Patients as Responsible Citizens. This attitude is extremely important for staff to adopt in order to work effectively with patients as well as with the community. The staff must believe that the people they are working with are citizens of the community; that they are living in the community because they have a right to and not because the community, through its good graces and kindness, is allowing them to be there; that they are indeed free agents able to make decisions and be responsible for their actions. These attitudes influence clinical behaviors. Take, for example the medication issue. The young adult chronic patient is frequently ambivalent about taking medications. We find we get better compliance if we relate to patients as responsible and make them partners in the medication decisions. We are willing to negotiate about dosage, we are willing to set a range within which patients control their own dosages dependent on how they perceive their needs. This approach makes them a part of the treatment process and treats them as responsible persons.

Another important clinical reason to treat patients as responsible is that many of them have learned that illness is an excuse for their behavior. We disabuse our patients of that notion. We tell them that indeed we believe that they are ill, otherwise we would not be prescribing medication, but that we do not believe their illness is an excuse for their behavior. We tell them that we will do everything we can to see to it that their positive behaviors are rewarded, but also that we will do our best to see to it that their negative behaviors get the same consequences that we would receive had we behaved that way. For example, we had one patient who would want to be rehospitalized whenever he became stressed and anxious. His way of doing that would be to go into a supermarket, take some soda and candy, and walk through the line without paying for it. If he was not apprehended, he would simply walk back in and load up some more until someone called the police. He would then get into the police car and half a block down the road would say to the policeman, "Oh, by the way, I'm a patient at Mendota State Hospital." At this point the policeman would sigh with relief, turn the car sharply to the left, and give him a free taxi ride out to the hospital. The policeman not only thought he was doing a good thing; he also avoided having to take him downtown, book him, write a detailed report, show up in court, and so on. To avoid the problem of the police taxiing the patient to the hospital, we had to work very closely not only with the police but with the district attorney and the judges to see to it that this kind of minor crime was handled as it would be for any other citizen. The next time this patient shoplifted at a supermarket he indeed went before a judge; the judge gave him the stern lecture he gives to all first offenders. The judge told him that "if you ever do this again you will spend three days in the county jail or have a $50.00 fine." For most patients that was enough, but a few patients had to find out if indeed the judge meant what he said. Thus after the second shoplifting event they went before the judge and they did get three days in the county jail or a $50.00 fine, and since they didn't have $50.00, proceeded to spend three days in the county jail. Our staff spent a good deal of that three days in the jail working not only with the patient but with the jailers to make sure everyone got through the three days all right. We found that, with this approach, the noted maladaptive coping with stress dropped precipitously. We are not advocating using this approach for people who break the law who are in the midst of a psychotic episode. We must use good clinical judgment to determine when this approach should be used. We have little difficulty in determining when our patients are consciously breaking the law as a maladaptive coping strategy and when they are doing things because they are really out of touch with reality.

Crisis Intervention Available Twenty-Four Hours a Day. This is a necessary part of a program when working with this group of patients. These patients don't limit their crises from nine to five, and hospital admissions generally are overrepresented after five at night, weekends, and on the holidays — periods of time when the normal support system is unavailable. Twenty-four hours per day availability of a crisis response ensures that a support system is always available to the patient. An important spinoff benefit of our crisis team is that it has markedly reduced hospitalization and thus has saved our system hundreds of thousands of dollars a year in inpatient costs. Those saved dollars are largely responsible for making it possible to operate our other community based programs.

Working with the Community

Providing support to community members who are in contact with our patients such as family members, landlords, storekeepers, agencies, and so on is just as important as working with the patient himself. These community members' attitudes about and modes of relating to patients are significant factors in influencing how well our patients do. The following are the principles we use in working with the community.

An Assertive Approach. Just as appropriate assertiveness is crucial in working with patients, it is also crucial in working with the community. For example, if one lets things slide with a landlord or an agency to the point where the decision has been made to evict or terminate the patient, it is then usually too late to repair the problem. The patient is extruded from that situation and the results of that extrusion are not only stressful to the patient but create a great deal of work for your staff. The solution is to closely monitor the relationship that your patient is having with the community he or she is in contact with, and to intervene early when difficulty presents itself.

Utilization of a Wide Variety of Community Resources. There are many public agencies that advertise themselves as providing services to the citizens of the community, but never contemplated they would be asked to provide those services to psychiatric patients. We recommend taking advantage of those agencies and getting them to provide services to psychiatric patients. Let us give two examples. One is the Visiting Nurse Service (VNS). The VNS a number of years ago in Dane County had virtually no psychiatric patients on the caseload. At the present time about 25 percent of their caseload are psychiatric patients. They give many of our prolixin injections; they visit patients in their homes; they serve an important monitoring function (if you really want to know how a patient is doing, visit his home and see how he is functioning there). Thus, the VNS has become a tremendous asset to us.

When we first approached them they were not jubilant about doing what they are now quite happy to do. They said, "We really don't know much about treating psychiatric patients and will probably do them more harm than good. Our staff doesn't have the proper training." We said in return that we understood that and would have one of our staff members accompany one of their staff members until their staff felt comfortable without our presence. They agreed and we gave them the support they needed. Now none of our staff members have to be with the Visiting Nurse Service. An added bonus is that the VNS has become a strong advocate for community treatment. We have had the same experience with other agencies who have not had prior experience with this population. Once they get to know and serve the population they become important advocates for the community treatment of that population. The explanation is quite simple, when agency workers get to know the patients and work with them over a period of time, they come to know patients as people; prior prejudices or myths that they might have had evaporate.

Let us give you one more example because it was one with which we had a difficult time. There is an agency that advertises itself as teaching home-making skills to the citizens of the community. We went to that agency and told them that we had a group of citizens who could use some of their help, and we further told them that these citizens had a psychiatric disability. They told us what we expected to hear: their staff had no experience with psychiatric patients and would probably do them more harm than good. We tried our standard approach by telling them we understood how they felt but would offer as much support as they needed, including having our staff members accompany theirs until they were comfortable enough to operate without them. They still refused. We then called their attention to the fact that they were a United Way agency and that the United Way had a rule that their agencies could not discriminate on the basis of disability. They advised us that they would be willing to take their chances with that, since not a very large part of their budget came from United Way. We then told them that the City of Madison had an ordinance which prohibited discrimination based on disability and that, if they continued to refuse, we would take them to court. It was at that point that they reluctantly agreed to work with our patients. The ending of that story is another happy one in that, given sufficient support, their staff indeed became comfortable with our patients, with a similar result to the one noted for VNS.

This second example makes the point that, if one is truly interested in getting the community to work with and accept these patients, there are times when one has to be willing to go the full route. It is difficult for any staff to go the full route unless they truly believe that these patients have a right to these services, a right to live in the community, and that the staff does not have to feel humbly grateful to the rest of the community for allowing patients to be there. It is absolutely crucial that your staff deeply believe that your patients are full citizens of the community and have the rights of all citizens. You must feel this to the depth of your soul so that you are imbued with the appropriate values that will help motivate you to instill those values in both your patients and in the community. We would like to emphasize that agency cooperation is not gotten by simply demanding it. It is necessary that your staff provide sufficient support in order to gain agency cooperation.

Providing Support and Education to Community Members. In addition to agencies, it is important to provide support and education to families, to landlords, to shopkeepers, and to whomever your patient comes into contact with. Rather than attempting to mount a mass education program we decided to educate and support community members every time there was a problem between a patient and a community member. For example, if we learned that one of our patients was having trouble with a shopkeeper, we would get together with the shopkeeper and do several things. First, we would teach the shopkeeper to relate to our patient in a very straightforward and unambiguous manner. After teaching him how to relate to our patients, we would use the event as an opportunity to teach about chronic mental illness. We would give the shopkeeper a realistic appraisal of that particular patient's dangerousness as well as the fact that chronic mentally ill people are no more dangerous than a random selection of the general population. We would then help him understand why a community based approach made more sense than institutional care, and we would emphasize that, although we might not approve of some of their behaviors, as good citizens we must be willing to tolerate nonlawbreaking, deviant behavior. Finally, we would leave the shopkeeper our card with our name and phone number on it and urge him to call us any time, twenty-four hours a day, seven days a week, if he experienced any problems or questions relating to our patiens. We found that providing this kind of education and support has led to greater community acceptance of our patients.

Retaining Responsibility for Patient Care. Coordination of the many services required by this patient population is necessary to a well-functioning community support system. In the past, we in mental health relied on referral and interagency communication as the means to attain coordinated services. This did not work; services frequently were poorly coordinated and incomplete. Although referral and interagency communication are necessary, they are not sufficient; the keystone to coordinated services is a fixed point of responsibility so that, even though there are many agencies providing services, one remains responsible to see that all those services are delivered (Test, 1979). The case manager model was developed to do that job. There are a number of different case manager models; we like and use the team case management model which we feel has several advantages for both patients and staff.

In addition to ensuring coordination, retaining responsibility for patient care means that a patient is not transferred or expelled from one program until he is well connected with another. We are sure you all have patients who tax your limits, and the decision is made that you can no longer work with that patient. We have a firm rule in our system that we cannot terminate with a patient until he is well connected with another program. If we cannot find another program, we continue to work with the patient until we do. Retaining responsibility also means we recognize many of our patients have lifelong disorders which require lifelong help. Thus, we make a commitment for life to a patient. The amount of service we may give during that lifetime varies tremendously. Some patients do so well that all they need is a phone call once a month just to find out how they are doing. Other patients require much more, and for most patients the amount of input varies over time. To operate as efficiently as possible we try to give the patient just what he needs; when he needs it, and where he needs it. In summary, retaining responsibility is crucial and it means ensuring that there is good agency coordination, that patients are not dropped from programs, and that treatment continues as long as the patient requires it.

Working with the Family. We believe the families of our patients have carried a double burden for too long a period of time (Lamb and Oliphant,

1979). They have carried the burden of having a member of their family stricken with a severe and chronic illness, and unfortunately, they have had to further cope with mental health professionals telling them that they were responsible for that illness: that the mother is schizophrenogenic; or the father is schizophrenogenic; or that the husband/wife relationship is pathological and resulted in producing a schizophrenic child; or that the whole family is sick and that the "identified patient" is carrying everyone's pathology so that the rest of them could be well. Although these theories are interesting they are post hoc and have very little data to support them. We do not think we are helping anybody, either the patient or the patient's family, by making them feel guilty or responsible for the illness. If the family is feeling guilty, working with them or with the patient is much more difficult. Cooperation of the family is frequently crucial in working with the young adult chronic patient and family guilt markedly reduces cooperation. Often it is useful to separate the patient from his family, which is difficult to do in any case, but almost impossible to do if the family is made to feel guilty. When working with families we do the following: (1) We do our best to try to persuade them that we do not hold them responsible for the illness. (2) We try to assess whether it is useful for the patient to continue to live at home with the family (Greenley, 1979; Leff, 1976). In some cases separation is a good thing and in some cases it clearly is not. We use family emotional overinvolvement, family criticality, and family intolerance as indicators as to whether to do a constructive family separation. (3) Whether we separate patients from their families or not, we continue to work closely with families. Providing support to the family frequently is as important as providing support to the patient.

Summary

The present generation of young adult chronic patients is the first generation of the postdeinstitutionalization movement patients. This is a group of patients that has spent, relatively speaking, little time in the hospital. They are difficult to work with for many reasons, and they tax the system quite heavily. How we develop treatment programs for them and how successful these programs are may have an enormous influence on how future services for future generations of patients will be designed.

References

Allen, P. "Response: A Consumer Perspective." *Proceedings of the Conference, Community Living Arrangements for the Mentally Ill and Disabled: Issues and Options for Public Policy.* Washington, D.C.: National Institute for Mental Health, 1976.

Greenley, J. R. "Family Symptoms, Tolerance, and Rehospitalization Experience of Psychiatric Patients." In R. G. Simmons (Ed.), *Research in Community and Mental Health.* Greenwich, Conn.: JAI Press, 1979.

Lamb, H. R., and Goertzel, V. "Discharged Mental Patients — Are They Really in the Community?" *Archives of General Psychiatry,* 1971, *24,* 29-34.

Lamb, H. R., and Oliphant, E. "Parents of Schizophrenics: Advocates for the Mentally Ill." In L. I. Stein (Ed.), *New Directions for Mental Health Services: Community Support Systems for the Long-Term Patient,* no. 2. San Francisco: Jossey-Bass, 1979.

Leff, J. P. "Schizophrenia and Sensitivity to the Family Environment." *Schizophrenia Bulletin,* 1976, *2,* 566–574.

Stein, L. I., and Test, M. A. "Alternative to Mental Hospital Treatment." *Archives of General Psychiatry,* 1980, *37,* 392–397.

Test, M. A. "Continuity of Care in Community Treatment." In L. I. Stein (Ed.), *New Directions for Mental Health Services: Community Support Systems for the Long-Term Patient,* no. 2. San Francisco: Jossey-Bass, 1979.

Turner, J. E. C., and Shifren, I. "Community Support Systems: How Comprehensive?" In L. I. Stein (Ed.), *New Directions for Mental Health Services: Community Support Systems for the Long-Term Patient,* no. 2. San Francisco: Jossey-Bass. 1979.

Leonard I. Stein is professor of psychiatry, University of Wisconsin Medical School, Madison, Wisconsin and medical director of the Dane County Mental Health Center.

Mary Ann Test is associate professor in the School of Social Work, University of Wisconsin.

*Crisis intervention can be successfully accomplished with
the difficult, young adult chronic patient population
by adhering to well-established principles of assessment
and crisis treatment adapted specifically for this population.*

Crisis Intervention with
the Young Adult
Chronic Patient

James W. Flax

Crisis intervention is a very difficult activity to engage in successfully, particularly with the young adult chronic population who often present therapists with a myriad of complicated problems. For this reason, one must approach such crises with a disciplined conceptual framework and focused yet rigorous assessment.

Of the approximately 800 patients who were identified as young adult chronic in a recent Rockland County sample, about 30 percent had been seen last in the Crisis Unit. An unknown number had been seen once or recurrently on the Crisis Service in the past, but were no longer in treatment there. This patient group represents approximately 7 percent of the 3,000 patients seen in any given year. Their crises can be quite difficult to assess, and they present therapists with so many problems in their management that they consume a far higher proportion of staff time than 7 percent.

A certain number of these patients resist or refuse ongoing and comprehensive treatment plans and have contact with our system only when they are intoxicated, suicidal, violent, psychotic, or otherwise in crisis. Others are regularly or sporadically in treatment, but nonetheless repeatedly visit the Crisis Unit (Bassuk and Gerson, 1980).

B. Pepper, H. Ryglewicz (Eds.). *New Directions for Mental Health Services: The Young Adult Chronic Patient*, no. 14. San Francisco: Jossey-Bass, June 1982.

Definition of Crisis

One definition commonly accepted for a crisis is Caplan's (1964):

The essential factor influencing the occurrence of crisis is an imbalance between the difficulty and importance of the problem and the resources immediately available to deal with it. The usual homeostatic, direct problem solving mechanisms do not work, and the problem is such that other methods which might be used to sidestep it also cannot be used. . . . Therefore, tension due to frustration of need rises, and this in itself involves problems in maintaining the integrity of the organism or group and may be associated with feelings of subjective discomfort or strain. A greater or lesser area of functioning is interfered with according to the intensity and significance of the problem and the strain. The individual is "upset." This upset is usually associated with such subjective feelings of displeasure as anxiety, fear, guilt, or shame, according to the nature of the situation. There is a feeling of helplessness and ineffectuality in the face of the insoluble problem, and this is associated with some disorganization of functioning, so that the person appears less effective than he usually is.

On our Crisis Unit we believe that this definition applies to young adult chronic patients as well as to any patient who may appear in a crisis. Although the young adult chronic patient's baseline level of functioning may be very different, and although the stressors precipitating their crisis — loss of a job, loss of a room, a quarrel with parents or with a friend — may be more frequent and, to the observer, more minor than the stressors precipitating crisis in our other patients, they are in crisis.

Our young adult chronic patients differ from our typical crisis patient in another way. They generally do not have a repertoire of adaptive coping mechanisms to draw upon, and their maladaptive mechanisms tend to be less socially acceptable and more extremely dysfunctional — including, for example, violent behavior, suicidal threats or gestures, and the development of delusions or hallucinations. The ego deficits which are observable to a lesser degree in their usual functioning — deficits in impulse control, reality testing, insight, judgment — make them vulnerable to major disorganzation in circumstances which, to our other patients, might present merely a difficult but common problem of everyday life. If we think in terms of Erik Erikson's (1963) concept of life as a series of developmental crises, we can see that, for most people, a developmental crisis associated with a transition in the life cycle commonly is resolved and followed by a long period of fairly stable functioning. We see our chronic young adult patients in the community as struggling repeatedly with developmental and functional tasks, often with increasingly ineffective means of coping, and rarely with a resolution leading to equilibrium.

A crisis is not merely an emergency. A young adult may come in with an extrapyramidal reaction to antipsychotic medication; that is an emergency but not necessarily a crisis. A crisis is produced by a hazardous event or a series of hazardous events—intrapsychic, biologic, social, environmental—superimposed upon a vulnerable state and it requires a straw to break the camel's back, a precipitating factor. This precipitating factor leads to a series of attempts at coping which, if unsuccessful, results in a crisis and perhaps major disorganization, and which may lead, in turn, to reorganization at an improved level. Crisis is in this sense an opportunity (Jacobsen, 1978, 1980). For our young adult chronic patients, the issue is often whether the crisis will lead to increasing dependence on hospitalization, to violent acting out, or to drug use as attempted coping behaviors, or to improved self-awareness and increased willingness to draw upon potential sources of support.

Assessment of the Patient in Crisis

In crisis intervention, the therapist is generally constrained by practical time limits. Thus, one must be efficient in the generation of hypotheses, ignoring extraneous information, and actively pursuing lines of questioning related to the patient's present crisis. In assessing the young adult chronic patient in crisis, we must rely not on the traditional intake method of gathering an exhaustive history but on the generation of hypotheses based on our initial observations in the first five or ten minutes (Lazare, 1981; Burgess and Lazare, 1976). The generation of hypotheses requires the use of a combination of theories that all potentially fit a particular patient. We have to avoid looking through one theoretical lens, because in doing so we may miss some very important data. If we look only through a biologic lens, we will try only biologic interventions and may miss three-quarters of the picture. Our hypotheses are partial formulations addressing a part of the clinical picture. We must employ all the lenses to generate enough hypotheses to flesh out the entire picture of the patient in crisis.

Case Example. A case examined in detail may illustrate this approach to assessment. Julie is a twenty-five-year-old black woman who has lived alone for the past nine months in the apartment portion of a single-family home. During these months, she has worked as a clerk in a large corporate headquarters. She was sent home from work on a Tuesday because her thinking had been confused and she was unable to function at her job. She felt that television and radio programs were directed specifically at her, believing that announcers were addressing her personal problems over the air. This was both reassuring and frightening to her.

Julie was socially withdrawn, having cut off contact from her two close friends and from all her large family except a brother. She came to the Crisis Unit with her brother, whom she had contacted for help. She had a history of three hospitalizations in the past four years, two of them at our facility. Until six weeks prior to this crisis, she had been seen on a monthly basis and given medication, having refused any other contact. Six weeks earlier she had decided to discontinue both her visits and her medication, trying to "make it on my own." At the time of her initial evaluation she was urged to come into the hospital, which she refused. Since she was not suicidal and was quite cooperative otherwise, the examining psychiatrist decided to attempt crisis intervention on an outpatient basis. He urged her to further involve her family, which she refused to do (Vaughn and Leff, 1981). She was encouraged to return for crisis intervention the following day, which she did.

What hypotheses might we consider in this case? A psychodynamic hypothesis can be based on knowledge of the precipitating event and its dynamic meaning for the patient. In Julie's case, she had attempted to be independent; working was very important to her, and being sent home from work was an event which dissolved her sense of independence. This, for her, was the crisis. Another psychodynamic hypothesis might be that this is a developmental crisis: She had attempted to separate from her parents and family, to individuate. She had wanted to see herself as independent and healthy but because of recent events was no longer able to do so. A sociocultural hypothesis might be that lack of social support facilitating movement toward her goals had left Julie in a vulnerable state.

A biologic synthesis would suggest that she was suffering from a nonaffective functional psychosis. In this regard, Julie's recent discontinuance of medication may be significant. Another biologic hypothesis — not confirmed in Julie's case but to be at least considered for almost any young adult chronic patient — would be that her problem resulted from the abuse of alcohol or other drugs.

In Julie's case, the developmental hypothesis did not appear especially illuminating. Data concerning her past hospitalizations with a diagnosis of schizophreniform disorder suggests that a biologic and sociocultural interpretation was more fruitful. Julie was suffering from a schizophrenic illness, aggravated by her decision to terminate medication. Cutting herself off from an already meager social support system was the precipitating factor of her crisis.

The Alliance. Whatever hypotheses we select in assessing a crisis — the most probable, the most serious, the most indicative of problems easily treated, or the most readily accepted by the patient — the hypotheses are always subject to revision. We cannot wait for all the facts before proceeding with treatment; diagnosis, therefore, permeates all stages of crisis intervention. We try, above all, to create a working alliance with the patient, which is crucial, of course, to voluntary outpatient treatment. This is what Aron Lazare (1981) refers to as the "customer approach to patienthood."

Two research observations which are germane to the crisis intervention setting support the importance of this working alliance. Gerson (1979), studying the determinants of hospitalization in an emergency room in Boston, has pointed out that when the customer approach was less feasible or less likely to be used, it was more likely that the patient would be hospitalized. Lambert (1979, p. 113) established a link between positive motivation and positive outcome. Motivation was viewed as "not only an interest in changing but a desire to change in ways that are congruent with the goals and values of the therapist." And the therapist, in my view, must relate his or her goals and values to those of the patient as well.

We must note that these elements of communication and motivation, based on shared values and understanding of the problem, are precisely what are lacking in many of our young adult chronic patients in crisis. The patients' denial and common difficulties in achieving insight or exercising judgment frequently make it difficult or impossible to create or maintain a working alliance. In the case of Julie, whom John Sheets (see Chapter Two, this volume) would place in the higher-functioning subgroup of these patients, such an alliance was possible, based on her motivation and acknowledgment of her problem.

Requests. An alliance is achieved through a process of negotiation, based on the patient's own request for help (Burgess and Lazare, 1976; Lazare, 1981). Julie's requests were for (1) *advice* — she wanted to know what to do about her job and about her delusions; (2) *clarification* — she wanted to take an active role in her treatment, which was consistent with her view of herself as an independent, functioning adult; and (3) *reality testing* — she wanted someone to reassure her that her delusions were not real, and to explain to her what they were.

These requests differ from the chief, or presenting, complaints and from the patient's goals. Julie's complaints were of being discharged from work, her confusion and sleeplessness, and her delusions. Her goal was to be well enough to return to work. Her requests were for the kinds of help she wanted from the clinician in order to achieve the desired goal. Another patient might request medication, hospitalization, or intervention with an employer, landlord, or family member. The negotiation is a process of reconciling and combining the kinds of help the patient requests and the kinds of help the clinician finds appropriate to offer. To Julie's requests, I would add three other clinically indicated kinds of help: (1) control of her social withdrawal and her delusions, (2) medication to treat what I see as a biologic illness, and (3) social intervention to address the breakdown in her social network.

Prerequisites for Outpatient Intervention

It is useful to consider the necessary conditions to carry out successful treatment of the psychotic young adult in an ambulatory setting (Bellak, 1978). First, there must be no signs of delirium in the psychotic patient. Second, it is very difficult to treat a first episode appropriately on an outpatient basis; it is much easier to do the necessary laboratory and medical workup on an inpatient unit, particularly when the patient is disorganized and psychotic.

Third, if a psychosis does not clear substantially with medication in the first four to six hours of observation, it is probably not suitable to attempt outpatient treatment. Fourth, if there is not continued remission after several days, then outpatient treatment is probably not feasible. Fifth, it requires a reasonably cooperative, nonassaultive patient who is not suicidal and is without severely disabling depression. Sixth, a patient needs to have a viable family or social support network — at least one stable relationship that offers someone to turn to in case of deterioration — or else a significant person who is provided by the treatment system (such as a case manager, an important element in our own system). Finally, it is necessary to have a close relationship with a nearby hospital as a precaution in case the patient's condition deteriorates.

In addition, an awareness of community resources can assist in restructuring the patient's day-to-day activities. Other necessary resources are a suitable housing situation; an emergency center with a twenty-four-hour hotline; an alarm system in your office, as these patients can be dangerous; and drug therapy combined with psychotherapy to stabilize the patient and enable psychosocial treatment to proceed. The importance of these various kinds of support cannot be stressed enough; they provide the setting that makes our work possible.

Julie returned to the clinic on an appointment basis and, after three days, we finally convinced her to begin taking the medication. She responded very quickly with rapid dissolution of her psychotic symptoms. At that point it was the Friday before a holiday weekend; she faced returning to a lonely apartment for three long days. We referred her instead to a crisis residence. The staff there ensured that she got her medication regularly and formed a strong relationship with her, helping her to plan for ongoing treatment. Ideally, a nonpathogenic family network is better. Lipton (1981), in a recent *Schizophrenia Bulletin*, gives data suggesting that the first hospital admission is the beginning of the dissolution of the patient's social network. Thus, the first break is a good time to intervene in order to preserve that network. But if, as in Julie's case, the family network is negative, it is best to help the patient separate by providing alternative supports.

Conclusion

Crisis treatment must consist of a diversified approach designed to decrease the patient's stress (Mendel, 1976). The approach must be timely and effective in order to establish a therapeutic alliance, if that is feasible. It must rescue the patient from pain and dysfunction before he or she is driven to possible suicide, and before the patient's social network becomes completely rejecting. Our job is to save patients from themselves, to avoid rewarding their symptoms and teaching them more symptoms, and to avoid providing lessons in how to be crazy. We avoid hospitalizing patients when possible, in order to discourage the use of hospitalization as a means of coping, and to keep other options alive. We seek alternative means of support, control, and environmental change through use of supportive families, the crisis residence, the day treatment program, or frequent contact with our own services. Julie utilized only some of our interventions, rejecting a referral to a day treatment program. She chose, instead, a week's "vacation" at the crisis residence, after which she was able to return to work and function on her job.

This was a successful crisis intervention with a relatively high-functioning young adult chronic patient, one to be followed by an ongoing treatment program (Herz, 1980). It illustrates one model for such intervention undertaken with one particular young adult chronic patient in our network of treatment resources.

References

Bassuk, E., and Gerson, S. "Chronic Crisis Patients: A Discrete Clinical Group." *American Journal of Psychiatry,* 1980, *137* (12), 1513–1517.

Bellak, L., and Small, L. *Emergency Psychotherapy and Brief Psychotherapy.* (2nd ed.) New York: Grune & Stratton, 1978.

Burgess, A. W., and Lazare, A. *Community Mental Health.* Englewood Cliffs, N.J.: Prentice-Hall, 1976.

Caplan, G. *Principles of Preventive Psychiatry.* New York: Basic Books, 1964.

Erikson, E. *Childhood and Society.* New York: Norton, 1963.

Gerson, S. "Determinants of Psychiatric Emergency Room Disposition." *Dissertation Abstracts International,* B 39(11) 5552 B, 1979.

Herz, M., and Melville, C. "Relapse in Schizophrenia." *American Journal of Psychiatry,* 1980, *137* (7), 801–805.

Jacobsen, G. "Crisis-Oriented Therapy." *The Psychiatric Clinics of America,* 1978, *2* (1), 39–54.

Jacobsen, G. F. (Ed.) *New Directions for Mental Health Services: Crisis Intervention in the 1980s,* no. 6. San Francisco: Jossey-Bass, 1980.

Lambert, M. J. "Characteristics of Patients and Their Relationship to Outcome in Brief Psychotherapy." In R. Sloane and F. Staples (Eds.), *The Psychiatric Clinics of North America. Symposium on Brief Psychotherapy.* Philadelphia: W. B. Saunders, 1979.

Lazare, A. *Outpatient Psychiatry, Diagnosis, and Treatment.* Baltimore: Williams and Wilkins, 1981.

Lipton, F. R., and others. "Schizophrenia: A Network Crisis." *Schizophrenia Bulletin,* 1981, *7* (1), 144–151.

Mendel, W. *Schizophrenia: The Experience and Its Treatment.* San Francisco: Jossey-Bass, 1976.

Pepper, B., Kirshner, M., and Ryglewicz, H. "The Young Adult Chronic Patient: Overview of a Population." *Hospital and Community Psychiatry,* 1981, *32* (7), 463–469.

Vaughn, C., and Leff, J. "Patterns of Emotional Response in Relatives of Schizophrenic Patients." *Schizophrenia Bulletin,* 1981, *7* (1), 43–44.

James W. Flax is a psychiatrist and the director of the Crisis Unit at the Rockland County Community Mental Health Center. He is also an assistant clinical professor of psychiatry at Columbia University.

A program of treatment by objectives focusing on identified problem areas is employed in a day treatment setting.

Treatment by Objectives: A Partial Hospital Treatment Program

G. G. Neffinger
J. W. Schiff

Over the past five years, a unique partial hospital unit has evolved at the Rockland County Community Mental Health Center called the Acute Day Treatment Program (ADTP). The ADTP consists of four service components. The Acute Stabilization component serves as an alternative to hospitalization. The Intensive Day Treatment (IDT) component provides transitional and supplemental partial hospital services (Neffinger, 1981). There is also a follow-up component called Extended Day Treatment (EDT), and an aggressive Medication/Monitoring Clinic.

The evolution of these services, as well as the unit's present organizational structure and general program offerings, are described in an earlier paper (Neffinger, 1980). This chapter will focus on the treatment philosophy and procedures followed in the Intensive Day Treatment and, to a lesser extent, the Extended Day Treatment segments of the program. Very briefly, IDT offers a fourteen-week, intensive, highly structured problem- and goal-oriented group-formulated program and milieu. EDT is a part-time, open-ended modification of Intensive Day Treatment.

Seventy percent of the ADTP population is under thirty, and a third of

B. Pepper, H. Ryglewicz (Eds.). *New Directions for Mental Health Services: The Young Adult Chronic Patient*, no. 14. San Francisco: Jossey-Bass, June 1982.

these have had two or more hospitalizations. Thus it should come as no surprise that a substantial number of ADTP clients could be classified as psychiatrically disabled young adults. The applicability and utility of the treatment program for this population will also be reviewed.

The treatment philosophy and derived procedures are referred to collectively as treatment by objectives, or TBO. This term is obviously and deliberately a take-off on the widely utilized planning and assessment system called management by objectives (MBO). MBO has three essential characteristics, which also describe its procedural steps: setting long-term or subordinate goals or objectives; setting of individual unit (person, department, and so on) goals by mutual agreement with the unit in question; and timely review and feedback of results, followed by another repetition of the entire protocol.

The basic idea is that "units" that clearly know and can articulate their objectives and have participated in the formulation of their goals and objectives will perform better (given access to appropriate means) and feel better about themselves than those who do not.

There is nothing radical about this proposal, although it was considered so when introduced by Peter Drucker (1954), the management guru. On examination, it turns out to be an explicit statement of an algorithm used by all good managers, and, at least to the extent of clear specifications of goals, is representative of the approach of all good problem solvers, whether they be engineers, managers, or psychotherapists. Since the role of the clinician in ADTP is to be a problem-solving resource person and trainer, the MBO technique as transformed into TBO seems like an obvious model upon which to base the treatment services at ADTP. The specific details of TBO follow.

Treatment by Objectives: The Process

Treatment by objectives is a multistep process involving a number of formal documents and procedures. In chronological order, as applied in IDT, they include general treatment goals in the intake interview, formal problem-area identification, and goal-of-the-week format. Their aim is to engage the client in a pragmatic approach to increasing adaptive and appropriate behavior preparatory to resuming a vocational and educational activity or work in the community.

At the time of the intake interview, a client is introduced to the philosophy and orientation of the program. The client's data base is openly reviewed. The interview then shifts to a concrete elaboration of the specific functional difficulties that the client perceives as treatment issues. Some of these areas are generally easy for the client to acknowledge, others are not. Arising out of this dialogue is a written contract, signed by the client, specifying a preliminary treatment plan, and also including a commitment to regular attendance and, if indicated, medication compliance and abstinence from substance abuse.

Within a week of admission, each client is asked to present a brief autobiography to the rest of the program community (clients and staff). This rein-forces the concept of group responsibility for planning and treatment. In addi-tion, it provides an opportunity for the client to publicly acknowledge his ini-tial treatment contract.

During their second or third week, problem area identification (PAI) takes place. The PAI procedure is based on a document which presents and defines thirty-five problem areas. These encompass four major areas of dys-function: general psychiatric symptoms (depression, disorientation, hallucina-tions), dysfunctional behavioral patterns (dependency, social skills deficits), specific role functioning (wage earner, parent or spouse), and pragmatic real-ity issues (living arrangement, legal and financial issues). The PAI procedure is conducted in the context of the individual's therapy group, which meets once a week in special session for this activity. Before this meeting takes place the target client has had a chance to study and review the PAI list and also to observe and participate in the PAI exercise for other clients.

In the PAI session the client is given the opportunity to present and explain the problem areas he has selected for himself. The rest of the group then becomes involved in editing the original list by both adding and subtract-ing problems. In this way, the client receives valuable direct feedback, both positive and negative, which both refines and clarifies the final list. The end result is a list of approximately six major problem areas or groupings of related problems as agreed upon both by the client and the rest of the group. The problem area list serves as the focus of treatment for the rest of the ADTP pro-gram for the client, although it can be expanded or contracted as circum-stances warrant.

In many cases, the PAI group is the first opportunity that a person has ever had to specifically delineate his areas of difficulty. Often there is a sense of relief that his problem is neither unique nor mysterious. Also, a commitment to work on the problem area is enhanced by this participatory development of the treatment plan. In those instances where problems are denied or resistance to treatment is a significant factor, the issue is addressed directly and immedi-ately, and possible reasons are explored. Other clients are encouraged to share their initial reactions and resistance.

The role of the therapist in treatment planning varies both with the level of dysfunction of the individual whose treatment plan is being formulated and the composition of the therapy group. In working with a verbal or treat-ment-experienced client, little intervention is needed. On the other hand, the group may have difficulty dealing with a client who presents himself as threat-ening or highly resistive. At that point the clinician assumes a more active role in dealing with the issue and in helping to formulate the final treatment plan. In no instance is the group uninvolved in this planning or is the plan formu-lated without the client's tacit consent. At the end of the exercise, the clinician combines the individual problem areas into groups reflecting highly correlated problems and speculates on which are primary and which are secondary. This is an educative process for all clients and encourages critical analysis of behavioral patterns and their significance.

The goal-of-the-week process is the heart of the TBO approach. A set of short-term goals, each keyed to a problem area, is established on a weekly basis. These goals are constructed in a progressive, hierarchical manner and constitute the treatment plan. That is, the weekly goals relate to the long-term goals, as a means to an end.

Each week every client is expected to present at least two short-term goals that he will accomplish in the following week. These goals, developed with staff input, must be concrete activities that relate directly to one or more problems the client has. They must pose at least a minimal challenge and must be objectively measurable. These goals are reviewed and the following week's goals presented at the regular group therapy session once each week. A formal goal sheet is maintained for each client which provides an ongoing log of the client's progress.

For clients, the goal of the week provides immediate positive reinforcement for specific adaptive behaviors. The acknowledgment of successfully completed goals is individual, as the client recognizes his own achievement; it is staff-initiated as the positive acknowledgment occurs during the individual goal conference; and it is public as the previous week's goals are reviewed in the therapy group. The process of partitioning the job to be done and providing a definite time frame is a unique aspect of the TBO format. It reduces unwieldy or threatening objectives to manageable and quantifiable tasks within the grasp of the client. This increases the probability for success with individuals discouraged by long-term failures.

As a streamlined example of TBO, take a client who has (among others) identified the problem areas of depression and vocational planning needs. The long-term goals, which are in effect the converse of these problems, are to have a positive self-image and optimistic outlook, and to have a clearly defined vocational plan which is in the process of being implemented. The initial short-term goal geared toward alleviating a retarded depression would be to have the client interact socially with at least one other client for ten minutes a day. The second week the interaction would be increased to twenty minutes daily and the client would eat lunch with other clients at least twice. In the case of an agitated depression, the client would start by listening to a tape on relaxation techniques (available on the unit) at least twice in the upcoming week. In the second week, the frequency of listening to the tape is increased to three times and the client is asked to practice the techniques at home on two separate occasions for twenty minutes each. In the third week, the client begins to read a book about dealing with self-denigrating thoughts. Reading successive chapters and completing successive exercises in the book become goals of the week over the next several weeks. Medication compliance, talking about oneself spontaneously in group therapy, and making positive self statements in conversation with other clients are additional goals aimed at reducing depression. As soon as the client is able to interact spontaneously in group and in other program activities as demonstrated by successful completion of the weekly goals (usually by the fifth week), the focus shifts to social interactions outside of program time, such as going to the movies with a family member and then with a friend. Further socialization goals are then added.

In a similar vein, vocational deficits are addressed in a graded series of tasks. The client begins by talking about his or her future plans and options in group therapy. The next goal is to make and keep an appointment with the vocational rehabilitation counselor. Subsequent weekly goals are then set with the help of the vocational counselor and include interest and aptitude testing, independent exploration and researching of economically and educationally feasible jobs, attending a weekly vocational group, checking course offerings and admission guidelines for the chosen field, making the application, and arranging financial aid.

Extended day treatment is designed as a follow-up and less intensive program. It incorporates many TBO components and is utilized primarily by psychiatrically disabled young adults. EDT consists of a half-day program, built around a one-and-a-half-hour group therapy session, that meets three times per week. There is no specific time limit, but clients are expected to be actively, substantially, and regularly engaged in some training program or paid or volunteer work in order to maintain their enrollment. In addition, a modified goal-attainment scaling procedure is used over six-week contract periods (Kiresuk and Sherman, 1968). Adequate goal attainment is also a condition of continued enrollment.

Assessment

In overview, TBO has several important characteristics that account for both its vitality and utility. The first of these is that it postulates a structure for both the clinician and the client. The external structure of program activity has as its counterpart the internal structure of treatment goals. The second characteristic is that of the explicit definition of problems and proposed solutions. Having a set of specific issues defined as the problem, related to a set of activities called goals designated as potential solutions, offers clients a rational framework from which to view and deal with the cataclysmic upheaval in their lives.

A third critical aspect of TBO is its time frame. The fourteen-week IDT period is not arbitrary. It reflects both the current literature on partial hospitalization length of stay and the data collected in a smaller pilot program. It is the combination of the explicit problem and goal treatment process with that of the time limitation which makes ADTP unique and successful as a demonstration project (Neffinger, 1980).

The ADTP clientele is generally young and nonchronic in the historical sense of the term. However, as mentioned earlier, a substantial minority of the clients, some with, but some without, prior hospitalizations are psychiatrically disabled young adults suffering from a major mental illness (schizophrenia, major affective disorder) or severe behavioral excesses or deficits of nonpsychotic types. These represent fully one-half of ADTP readmissions, which themselves represent approximately 25 percent of total admissions in any given time period. The percentage of psychiatrically disabled young adults in the program at any given time ranges from 5 to 40 percent.

The psychiatrically disabled young adult client arrives at the ADTP with a long history of failures: functional, social, and vocational. Low self-esteem and the inability to recognize or acknowledge accomplishments are often concomitants to this picture. TBO begins to build a pattern of success by gearing each weekly goal to the client's current functioning level. With each completed task, a pattern of success is initiated and the client is encouraged to validate his own accomplishment, so that approval becomes internalized as well as external.

In general, the psychiatrically disabled young adults have done well with TBO. The elements of the program which they report as most helpful are the community spirit, the structure, and the goal focus. This is particularly true of the readmitted clients who have often drifted through the program in a sealing-over (Aiello, 1979) or pure socialization mode on their first admission. The second and even the third time, they are more highly motivated and deliberately choose to be referred to ADTP with full appreciation of the demands that will be made and the effort that will need to be expended. These individuals usually adopt an integrative approach to their disability (Aiello, 1979) and seek to revitalize and practice social skills and so some serious future vocational and life-style planning.

Although TBO's inherent flexibility and its capacity for individual fine tuning makes it infinitely adaptable, it is clear that it has not met all the needs of the psychiatrically disabled young adults. Two drawbacks are obvious. First, TBO typically seems to fail, as do most therapeutic endeavors, when motivation for change is at an ebb. This lack of motivation is not the same as despondency, but rather a resignation to accept life at a suboptimal level. Often these clients are chronic sealing-over types. They also present with significant substance abuse (alcohol or pot), which is an obvious self-medicating behavior. They are the impervious whom neither seduction nor threat can reach. A second specific drawback of TBO for the treatment of the psychiatrically disabled young adult is the fourteen-week time limit. This is the one element about which the psychiatrically disabled young adult client most frequently complains. These complaints seem clinically justified.

These considerations suggest that a program designed specifically for psychiatrically disabled young adults should include (1) a firm yet flexible structure, (2) a low-key problem and goal orientation, (3) open-ended participation, and (4) a deliberately and assiduously cultivated social milieu extending beyond the physical and temporal boundaries of the program. The extended day treatment component represents a deliberate effort to incorporate these programming elements in order to meet the need of the psychiatrically disabled young adult.

TBO is not, therefore, an answer to how to treat the psychiatrically disabled young adult. It was never designed to be either syndrome- or cohort-specific; it was designed as a flexible, adaptable treatment philosophy and method within the community mental health mode. Nevertheless, it is perhaps, in its most liberal version, a good first approximation for the definitive treatment of the psychiatrically disabled young adult.

References

Aiello, J. J. "Short-Term Group Therapy of the Hospitalized Psychotic." In H. Grayson (Ed.), *Short-Term Approaches to Psychotherapy*. New York: Human Sciences Press, 1979.

Drucker, P. *The Practice of Management*. New York: Harper & Row, 1954.

Humble, J. W. *How to Manage by Objectives*. New York: AMACOM, 1973.

Kiresuk, T. J., and Sherman, R. E. "Goal Attainment Scaling: A General Method for Evaluating Comprehensive Mental Health Programs." *Community Mental Health Journal*, 1968, *4*, 443–453.

Neffinger, G. G. "The Evolution of an Acute Day-Treatment Program." *Hospital and Community Psychiatry*, 1980, *31*, 826–828.

Neffinger, G. G. "Partial Hospitalization: An Overview." *Journal of Community Psychology*, 1981, *9*, 262–269.

G. G. Neffinger is the primary architect and present director of the Acute Day Treatment Program at Rockland Community Mental Health Center. He holds the diplomate in clinical psychology from the American Board of Professional Psychology.

J. W. Schiff, ACSW, is the senior psychiatric social worker at the Acute Day Treatment Program.

A growth advancement program (GAP) designed specifically for
young adults employs a combination of group and activity therapy.

GAP: A Treatment Approach
for the Young Adult
Chronic Patient

Miriam Schacter
William Goldberg

The emergence of a group of chronically ill young adults in the community has
been documented within the past year by several observers (Bassuk and Gerson, 1980; Schwarz and Goldfinger, 1981). Talbott (1981, p. 47) notes that
the large number of post-World War II babies are now at the age when they
are most likely to develop schizophrenic and other chronic or episodic psychiatric conditions. Simultaneously, concern about the effects of long-term institutionalization and legal restraints on involuntary admissions had led to the
necessity of treating these young adults in the least restrictive setting. As Pepper, Kirshner, and Ryglewicz (1981) point out, this is the first generation of
chronic individuals to have to cope throughout their lives with the tasks and
stresses of community living. In this chapter, we shall describe a successful
treatment program for chronic young adults, the Rockland County Community Mental Health Center's Growth Advancement Program (GAP).

History of GAP

Since 1971, the Community Support Center had been treating clients
of a variety of ages and a cross section of diagnostic categories, all of whom

B. Pepper, H. Ryglewicz (Eds.). *New Directions for Mental Health Services: The Young Adult
Chronic Patient*, no. 14. San Francisco: Jossey-Bass, June 1982.

were in need of a full-time, long-term supportive day program. Between 1977 and 1979, the agency integrated a large number of older chronic schizophrenic, institutionalized individuals. The Community Support Center adapted to the changing needs of this population and the program was no longer a viable option for the younger client who also needed long-term supportive treatment. The young adults who were referred to this program would often attend for one day, look around them at the middle-aged and elderly institutionalized clients, and refuse to return. Indeed, we viewed this refusal to become identified with the chronically ill deinstitutionalized population as a sign of health in the young adults. The Acute Day Treatment Program, a fourteen-week, structured, goal-oriented day hospital program, was not an adequate option, since its focus was upon rapid reintegration of acutely ill individuals back to the community and not upon providing a long-term program for chronically ill individuals (see Chapter Nine, this volume). Simultaneously, the outpatient mental health clinics found themselves dealing with a young adult population who were not benefitting from traditional individual or group psychotherapy. An inordinate amount of staff time was being consumed by these young adults, who were neither highly motivated nor introspective. These clients often cancelled appointments when they were not experiencing acute pain or anxiety, but would appear in the clinics during times of crisis and demand service. Clearly, these clients were in need of a different treatment modality. They required long-term care in a flexible, supportive environment with a staff able to respond to frequent crises.

The Growth Advancement Program (GAP) was created in August, 1979, as a response to this gap in service. The treatment modality utilized in GAP was based upon a group initiated two years previously at the Community Support Center for young adults whose primary need was to develop an adequate support system in the community. In addition to this problem, many of them were involved in destructive family relationships, did not have a consistent or constructive peer group, and were unable to maintain themselves on a job.

The group met in the evening to obviate the problem of mixing young adults and middle-aged clients. This group was co-led by a psychiatric social worker and a mental health worker, both of whom were part of the Community Support Center's staff. The group met for two hours once a week, spending their time either in group therapy, participating in a group activity, or, as was more often the case, a combination of the two. This combination proved to be an excellent treatment modality for overcoming fears and anxieties regarding social interaction. The group was able to engage in an activity within a protective environment with group workers who would encourage the participants to speak openly about their discomforts. This group proved to be a tremendous success, since individuals who were never able to utilize mental health services in the past were now becoming involved. The discovery of this successful treatment modality and the recognition of the service needs of the chronic young adult population led to the creation of the GAP program.

The primary focus of GAP is to encourage the participants to create a social system for themselves outside the agency. Group leaders actively encourage members to interact outside the group by identifying common areas of interest and by modeling appropriate social behavior. Another important focus of GAP is to encourage members to take an active role in their treatment by requiring that they accept joint responsibility for the group's use of time. In other words, each week the members themselves decide whether the group will focus upon a discussion, an activity, or a combination of both.

Subgroups Within the Young Adult Chronic Population

We have observed that individuals who can benefit from the GAP program fall into one of four categories and we have grouped them accordingly. These groups are differentiated by their members' capacity to contend with problems and by the fact that they struggle with slightly different issues.

The first group consists of young adults with either a diagnosis of schizophrenia or borderline personality disorder. All of them struggle with the issue of separation from their families. A few are able to take courses at a local community college. Some are able to maintain part-time employment on a sporadic basis. However, when they attempt to work, they tend to be overwhelmed by anxiety and to react to pressure by withdrawing or decompensating. As with the other groups, an overriding issue is their inabilty to maintain constructive peer relationships.

A second group consists of young adults who are both mentally retarded and emotionally disturbed. Most of them live with families, who tend to be overprotective. Others live in group homes. The members of this group are involved in either a sheltered workshop or work full time. All of them are socially isolated and are overwhelmed in an unstructured social situation.

A third group consists of young adults who are either mentally ill or have a primary diagnosis of learning disability. Like the members of the second group, most of these individuals live with their families, attend sheltered workshops or are employed, and have a major problem with peer relationships. The primary difference between these two groups is that the members of this group are better able to develop insight into their difficulties, since they are not developmentally disabled.

The combination of group therapy and activity therapy proved to be effective. A few months after GAP's inception, the program began to receive referrals of individuals who could benefit from this GAP program but who were not young adults. We therefore began an adult group for individuals aged thirty-five to fifty-five. As with the young adults, their primary need is to develop a support system for themselves in the community.

As GAP has become an established component of the Rockland County Community Mental Health Center, we have received a large number of referrals of individuals who are not able to benefit from the program's present structure. These young adults have difficulty concentrating on a task and thus are unable to become engaged either in school or work. They manifest a tremendous amount of rage and have not developed acceptable avenues for discharging this rage. They tend to stay home, sometimes remaining in bed most of the day, and become a management problem for their families. They have had a series of hospitalizations and tend not to follow through with assigned treatment plans. Their delusional systems are active and their use of recreational drugs is frequent. We are, therefore, establishing for this population an afternoon program with an emphasis on recreational therapy. Our goal is to lure these individuals from their homes and to help them become involved in constructive therapeutic group activities.

GAP Services and Staff

In addition to weekly group sessions, individual psychotherapy, family therapy, vocational counseling, and medication are offered to GAP clients when indicated. We emphasize the necessity of tailoring treatment services to meet individualized needs. To that end, we will accept clients into the GAP program who, upon admission, are unable to become part of a group. These clients are seen individually with the goal of eventually integrating them into a group while they continue their individual therapy. Similarly, we will accept clients into GAP groups without requiring them to immediately terminate with the referring therapist.

The GAP staff consists of a coordinator who, in addition to co-leading one of the groups, is administratively responsible for the program and clinically supervises the staff. Other staff members include a psychiatrist, a psychiatric nurse, four psychiatric social workers, two rehabilitation counselors, an art therapist, and two mental health workers. The coordinator and one rehabilitation counselor work full time for GAP while the remainder of the staff is assigned part time to GAP and part time to the Community Support Center day treatment program. This staff serves a caseload of ninety clients.

The fact that the GAP program is physically located in the Community Support Center building has proven to be a significant advantage because other Community Support Center staff can be called upon to integrate GAP clients into their program areas, particularly when a client is in crisis and in need of a structured day program. As previously mentioned, a difficulty with this intervention is that the young adults often become confused and angry when they are identified with the older chronic clients. In the near future, we plan to devote a wing of the Community Support Center Building entirely to the GAP program so that contact between these populations is minimized.

In addition to individual clinical supervision, the entire program staff meets for weekly group supervision. Group supervision has proven to be an effective tool in countering the inevitable feelings of frustration and burnout that are a concomitant of working with this population. These clients are frustrating, depressing, and sometimes frightening. In addition to discussing problematic issues, group supervision affords the staff the support and encouragement which they need. Also, because we utilize the group as the primary treatment modality in GAP, it has been helpful for the staff to meet in an ongoing group themselves. Continuity of care by the same treatment staff is crucial in establishing therapeutic alliances with this client population and the existence of a supportive group is one of the factors which has maintained staff consistency within the program.

The Growth Advancement Program, then, has proven to be an important component of service in working with the chronically mentally ill young adult. The combination of group therapy and activity therapy as well as the emphasis upon building a support system outside the group has had a significant impact upon individuals who were previously unable to sustain a constructive relationship with their peers. The Growth Advancement Program, along with case management, the crisis unit, the Acute Day Treatment Program, and the Inpatient Unit, has proven to be an effective treatment modality for this population.

References

Bassuk, E., and Gerson, S. "Chronic Crisis Patients: A Discrete Clinical Group." *American Journal of Psychiatry,* 1980, *137* (12), 1513-1517.
Pepper, B., Kirschner, M. C., and Ryglewicz, H. "The Young Adult Chronic Patient: Overview of a Population." *Hospital and Community Psychiatry,* 1981, *32* (7), 463-469.
Schwartz, S. R., and Goldfinger, S. M. "The New Chronic Patient: Clinical Characteristics of an Emerging Subgroup." *Hospital and Community Psychiatry,* 1981, *32* (7), 470-474.
Talbott, J. A. "Commentary." *Hospital and Community Psychiatry,* 1981, *32* (7), 447.

Miriam Schacter, ACSW, is coordinator of the Growth Advancement Program of the Rockland County Community Mental Health Center.

William Goldberg, ACSW, is program supervisor for rehabilitative services, Rockland County Community Mental Health Center.

Family crisis intervention on an inpatient unit can be
a point of departure for work in either a psychoeducational
or a family systems model.

Working with the Family of the Psychiatrically Disabled Young Adult

Hilary Ryglewicz

The subject of family intervention with the young adult chronic patient is one that induces a touch of professional schizophrenia. There is a dynamic tension in psychiatric theory and practice which sometimes, and regrettably, takes the form of a polarization. At one end we have the traditional medical model, in which the patient is identified without quotation marks and is seen as suffering from an illness, biogenetic in its origins, which clinicians try to treat and to help families to manage. At the other pole we have the family systems model, in which the disorderly thinking and behavior of identified patients is seen as integral to family structure and process, which are viewed as the proper focus of treatment. The model used tends, of course, to determine both how we speak and what we do. For some people who try to treat (or respond to) these difficult young adults, the family factor is almost an afterthought. For others, the family factor is really the whole.

Between these two poles there has been more of a meshing in practice than in theory. The importance of dealing with the family is as often acknowledged today as it is variously understood. But, dealing with it how, in what ways, and with what goals?

B. Pepper, H. Ryglewicz (Eds.). *New Directions for Mental Health Services: The Young Adult Chronic Patient*, no. 14. San Francisco: Jossey-Bass, June 1982.

New Directions for Mental Health Services: New Developments in Interventions with Families of Schizophrenics (1981) presented an array of programs directed primarily toward the reduction of relapse and rehospitalization rates through the reduction of expressed emotion (EE) levels in families including a schizophrenic member. These psychoeducational model programs feature a highly structured and intensive series of family interventions. They are combined with the use of psychotropic medications and in fact contribute to improved compliance with psychopharmacological and other treatment. As another, more comprehensive model, C. Christian Beels (1976) describes a program begun in the mid-1960s at what is now Bronx Psychiatric Center, based on a family and social systems model and designed "to do everything for its population, while providing continuity of care," recognizing that "the family and patient sense that their predicament may last a lifetime" (p. 257).

Both of these models of family intervention are readily applicable to a medically oriented treatment agency. Although the Bronx program obviously required a much broader and more ambitious level of support for family intervention, the psychoeducational programs have the advantage of being clearly limited in their goals, defined in detail in both their structure and their methods, and directly related to the growing edge of research into the course of schizophrenia (Anderson and others, 1981; Berkowitz and others, 1981; Brown and others, 1972; Falloon and others, 1981; Goldstein and Kopeikin, 1981; Snyder and Liberman, 1981).

How can we relate these models to our present concern with the young adult chronic patient? We commonly first meet the families of disturbed young people in an emergency room, a crisis service, or an inpatient unit. This chapter is an account of family intervention as it is practiced on the Rockland County Community Mental Health Center (RCCMHC) Inpatient Unit,* in a form that I believe can be generalized to the majority of treatment situations.

When we meet with the family of a seriously disturbed young adult, we are entering a field of powerful and conflicting emotional forces. Some parents first come to us after years of frustration and conflict with their young adult member. Others have suffered a sudden, heavy, and traumatic blow of a psychotic break in a seemingly well-functioning son or daughter. In either case, a family's reflex response is to ask why? — either "What have I (or we) done wrong?" or "Why is he or she doing this to us?" It is very difficult to keep the question of cause or causes from becoming an attempt to affix blame.

Our own quick suppositions about who is making whom crazy, and how, have been given substance by a great deal of clinically based theory,

*I am indebted to Dr. A. O. Stein of the Inpatient Unit at RCCMHC for both the enriching and instructive experience of participating in his work with families, and for much of my own awareness of what goes on, and what should go on, when patients, families, and staff sit down together.

nearly all of which has yet to be definitively confirmed by research (Liem, 1980). Our awareness of double-binding communications in the families of schizophrenics (and others) has been followed inescapably by the observation that parents, too, may confront classic double binds in interaction with their children. For parents of the young adult chronic patient, the primary injunction is: Take care of your child, and respond when he or she needs you. The secondary and conflicting injunction is: Do not treat your adult son or daughter as a dependent child, for you will then be feeding into the dependency. The third condition is that there is no exit; there is no escape in this life from being the parent. A parent, who may do a lot of bailing out or may turn away in seeming callousness, must still carry the burden of failed personal and social expectations.

The question of who drives whom crazy is unsettled as well as unsettling. So, too, is the question of how family dynamics and genetic predispositions interact, in what proportions, to produce the complex and sometimes blatant tragedies of family life for the psychiatrically disabled young adult. Meanwhile, many families are waiting at the door for our response to their torment. We have to meet them without definitive answers to the question of why?; and yet, we must manage to talk meaningfully with them about the presenting crisis as well as the long-term picture.

In a crisis, we know that we need to move as rapidly as possible to mobilize all resources; to clarify what has happened and what may be expected; to gather as much relevant background information as possible; and to offer enough reassurance to reduce anxiety to a level where it is no longer panic, but can be utilized to work toward change and mastery. On our inpatient unit, the family piece of the crisis intervention is handled in such a way that (1) the family is involved, at as early a stage as possible; (2) the problem is discussed in terms that, while admitting to what we do not know, are meaningful and valid regarding what we do know of etiology, prognosis, and management, and that put aside the impulse and need to place blame; (3) the seriousness of the problem and the uncertainties of prognosis are recognized and on the other hand, (4) possibilities for positive courses of action and potential growth are identified, including (5) realistic ways of handling the family relationships and issues as they are expressed in everyday situations, with information about (6) how we as professionals hope to be of help, and what resources we can offer, with a view toward (7) helping both the young adult and the family to develop resources outside their relationship, so that they can move in the direction of gradually letting go.

That sounds like a tall order. What does it mean in practice? First, to involve the family means communicating promptly, firmly and empathetically, first with the young adult patient about contacting the family, and then with the family directly.

Bringing about the first meeting often involves grappling with tremendous resistance. If we are determined to marshall all forces and gather all necessary understanding, the task is to get all the family together. This means gathering all members of the household, past or present, and significant other relatives who are involved with the patient. This in turn may mean parents whose home the young adult has already physically left; it may include siblings who have left the home; it may sometimes involve their coming from considerable distances, and sometimes bringing their husbands or wives. It may mean that involved grandparents come, or the sympathetic aunt to whom the young adult goes for refuge when the parents periodically throw him or her out. It may involve divorced parents sitting down together for the first time in years to confront the problems of their adult child. It may mean that quite young children in the family come and contribute valuable input, and perhaps have the opportunity to relieve their own anxieties through hearing open discussion of confusing events.

The process of setting up such a meeting is often itself very informative. The young adult may protest that he or she does not want to cause the parents any more trouble or heartache by asking them to come. One or the other parent, most commonly the father, may present himself as unavailable because of work responsibilities. The young adult may indicate that a sister or brother would not be interested and may gain support from learning that this is not the case. The parents may protest that the grandparents do not even know about the hospitalization, but have been told some palatable story, or that they hope the meeting will be without the young adult patient, because they wouldn't feel free to talk frankly in front of him; or that the children should not be dragged in to such a terrible place as a mental hospital; or that trying to talk about these problems with so-and-so (and this so-and-so may be a husband or wife with whom one is living) will lead to a fight.

These initial reactions are part of the process of getting to know a family; they offer clues to the relationships and issues within a family, and to how these may relate, if not to the etiology of the psychiatric disorder, at least to how the family impinges upon its course. To hold such a gathering also constitutes an intervention, an impinging of the treatment team's values upon the family system. It communicates quite a different message and yields quite different results from those of the traditional hospital practice of having the social worker take a history from one or both parents. Bringing together the family and the professional "family" of the treatment team offers an incomparable opportunity to carry out a number of purposes: to gather the fullest possible information, including interactions and differing perceptions of the problem; to open up communication within the family; to make a model for the frank acknowledgment and discussion of psychotic symptoms and not merely their management, but their possible secondary functions within the family system; and to set from the beginning the pattern of working together in such a way that all staff have direct knowledge of the family and are available as resources to family members.

Such meetings do not always go smoothly and calmly. People may shout and they may weep. The identified patient may walk out (usually to return later) or make a sudden move toward physical violence which has to be contained. While such emotional outbursts are not the goal of the meeting, nor are they encouraged, they may demonstrate to a family that it can survive them, or demonstrate to staff what has been happening at home, and they may clear the way for working toward understanding, acceptance, and change. Often people have to mourn or to rage about the disappointment and loss of their expectations before they can create more realistic expectations.

On our inpatient unit, a short-term, crisis oriented unit where the median stay is seventeen days, family meetings are generally held on a weekly basis while the identified patient remains in the hospital. The content and format of such meetings and the group's composition vary with the nature of the family, and with their capacity and willingness to pursue significant issues that relate to the young adult's developmental crisis and to that of the family system. With some families the work is limited to the sharing of information, discussion of prognosis, aftercare plans, and methods of coping with difficulties which arise in daily living. With others there may be an exploration and clarification of family history and relationships if such issues are current for the young adult patient. With still others the major focus may be on ground rules to be developed for the containment of a young adult's disruptive behavior, or to prevent his or her relapsing into apathy.

It is not infrequent in such family encounters to find that the parents are in severe marital conflict or emotional divorce, or that a parent or sibling is an untreated alcoholic and may be willing, in the crisis of the young adult's episode, to seek help or to identify younger children who are in dire need of treatment. In this regard, involvement of the family may serve a preventive or rehabilitative purpose which goes beyond the immediate response to the crisis of the young adult patient.

This approach to working with families of psychiatrically disabled young adults in the context of brief hospitalization is compatible with either a medical or a family systems model. It is founded on principles of crisis intervention rather than on a specific theory of family therapy or of the etiology of mental and emotional disorders. Through prompt initiation of involvement with the entire family, the way is opened for a flexible response to families with different capacities and needs, utilizing elements of the psychoeducational and family systems model as the situation permits or requires. This flexibility is doubly important in the setting of a small, short-term receiving hospital with a heterogeneous patient and family population, and also in view of our definition of the young adult chronic patient group in functional terms which cut across diagnostic lines. Elements of Haley's (1980) focus on restoration of the parental hierarchy and Lansky's (1977) idea of family responsibility for the handling of passes and timing of discharge are readily utilized in family sessions and in the operation of the unit.

The goals of this family crisis intervention are obviously limited by the fact that it is so crisis oriented and brief. Ideally, it is a first step, to be followed by an ongoing relationship with families, especially those with a severely and persistently dysfunctional young adult member. Families now can be referred, from Inpatient or elsewhere, to a multiple-family group recently initiated in our system.

Let us return, in conclusion, to the issue of terminology as it relates to contrasting models or ways of perceiving a young adult's psychiatric disorder. To describe a young person's difficulty as mental illness suggests one set of expectations; to identify his or her behavior as a response to tensions in a family system or as some kind of perversely goal-directed behavior suggests other expectations about who should do what toward whom, and why. Expectations are closely related to the roles in which people see each other and themselves. If the young adult and the parents see him or her in the role of dependent child or sick person, and the parents in the role of nurturers (as is appropriate for a child) or caregivers (as is appropriate for someone who is ill), the situation will remain static — unless room can be made for expectations that the child will progressively grow up or that the patient will eventually grow well. There is a hazard, then, in speaking of patients who are mentally ill, and if we go on to call them chronically disabled, however descriptive the term in our experience, we are taking the risk that, once we have modified our expectations and those of families so that no one will expect too much, not much will happen. Family systems theories of disorderly behavior such as Haley's tend to sound more optimistic. The hazard they create is perhaps that we may encourage an expectation of functioning that, for some individuals, is impossible, and may then blame our failures on families, on patients, or on ourselves.

What we need is to help families to expect enough, yet not too much. We can observe, for instance, that some families get into the position of being tyrannized by the needs and behavior of an explosive or withdrawn young adult. This may happen all the more readily if the patient is labeled sick. Other families may be insensitive to a young adult's mental illness or personality disorder and have overambitious or rigid expectations of behavior. Still other families may have difficulty allowing any room for growth in a chronically disabled young adult, but may instead present an attitude that is at once overanxious and critical; other families withdraw as much as possible from contact with a young adult they see as hopelessly disabled or as incorrigibly troublesome.

It would make sense, then, to place our emphasis, through the terms we use, on those aspects of a young adult's problems that are not acknowledged by the family, so that those who are tyrannized by their "sick" adult child may be encouraged to make reasonable demands and to set limits; and, hopefully, those who hold to over-demanding expectations may adopt an attitude of greater tolerance, based on their understanding of the young adult's disorder.

Beels (1976), writing about how to describe schizophrenia, says that "all ways of talking about it are metaphors . . . and we try to use metaphors that are as consistent, communicative, and truthful as possible. . . ." (p. 251). But he says, too, that "we need to go beyond our present individual diagnostic approach to the classification of patients, and instead to classify the lives of patients in family, economic, and treatment systems" (p. 279). The issue, after all, is not whether we believe in family therapy or in mental illness, but what metaphors and what actions will help a particular dysfunctional young adult to begin functioning, and how family interventions may contribute to that outcome.

References

Anderson, C. M., Hogarty, G., and Reiss, D. J. "The Psycho-Educational Family Treatment of Schizophrenia." In M. J. Goldstein (Ed.), *New Directions for Mental Health Services: New Developments in Interventions with Families of Schizophrenics,* no. 12. San Francisco: Jossey-Bass, 1981.

Beels, C. C. "Family and Social Management of Schizophrenia." In P. J. Guerin, Jr. (ed.), *Family Therapy: Theory and Practice.* New York: Gardner Press, 1976.

Berkowitz, R., Kuipers, L., Eberlein-Frief, R., and Leff, J. "Lowering Expressed Emotion in Relatives of Schizophrenics." In M. J. Goldstein (Ed.), *New Directions for Mental Health Services: New Developments in Interventions with Families of Schizophrenics,* no. 12. San Francisco: Jossey-Bass, 1981.

Brown, G. W., Birley, J. L. T., and Wing, J. K. "Influence of Family Life on the Course of Schizophrenic Disorders: A Replication." *British Journal of Psychiatry,* 1972, *121,* 241–258.

Falloon, I. R. H., and others. "Family Management Training in the Community Care of Schizophrenia." In M. J. Goldstein (Ed.), *New Directions for Mental Health Services: New Developments in Interventions with Families of Schizophrenics,* no. 12. San Francisco: Jossey-Bass, 1981.

Goldstein, M. J., and Kopeikin, H. S. "Short- and Long-Term Effects of Combining Drug and Family Therapy." In M. J. Goldstein (Ed.), *New Directions for Mental Health Services: New Developments in Interventions with Families of Schizophrenics,* no. 12. San Francisco: Jossey-Bass, 1981.

Haley, J. *Leaving Home: The Therapy of Disturbed Young People.* New York: McGraw-Hill, 1980.

Lansky, M. R. "Establishing a Family-Oriented Inpatient Unit." *Journal of Operational Psychiatry,* 1977, *8* (1), 66–74.

Leff, J. P. "Developments in Family Treatment of Schizophrenia." *Psychiatric Quarterly,* 1979, *51.*

Liem, J. H. "Family Studies of Schizophrenia." *Special Report: Schizophrenia 1980.* Washington, D.C.: National Institute for Mental Health, 1980.

Snyder, K. S., and Liberman, R. P. "Family Assessment and Intervention with Schizophrenics at Risk for Relapse." In M. J. Goldstein (Ed.), *New Directions for Mental Health Services: New Developments in Interventions with Families of Schizophrenics,* no. 12. San Francisco: Jossey-Bass, 1981.

Hilary Ryglewicz, ACSW, is clinical assistant to the director at the Rockland County Community Mental Health Center in Pomona, New York.

Effective and relevant programs for the newly identified service population of young adult chronic patients must be firmly rooted in the community's system of mental health services.

Program Planning for Young Adult Chronic Patients

Leona L. Bachrach

The purpose of this chapter is to try to bridge the gap between two trends: one, the increasing recognition of the young adult chronic patient population; and the other, the growth of so-called model programs for the care of chronically psychiatrically impaired individuals.

With regard to the first of these trends, that of the increasing recognition and understanding of young adult chronic patients — including both potential patients as well as those individuals who are actually enrolled in psychiatric facilities — we are still in a relatively early stage. However, thanks largely to the pioneering efforts of Bert Pepper in convening two conferences devoted to the study of this special population (Suffern, N.Y., November, 1980; and Albany, N.Y., June, 1981), and to several articles published recently on this subject (*Hospital and Community Psychiatry*, July, 1981; March, 1982), considerable attention is now being focused on these patients. The second trend — the growth of model programs for chronic mental patients — is of longer duration and can be viewed within the context of accumulated experience.

Although the problem of serving the young adult chronic patient is a

Adapted from an article, "Young Adult Chronic Patients: An Analytical Review of the Literature," by Leona L. Bachrach, *Hospital and Community Psychiatry*, March 1982, *33*, 189–197.

B. Pepper, H. Ryglewicz (Eds.). *New Directions for Mental Health Services: The Young Adult Chronic Patient*, no. 14. San Francisco: Jossey-Bass, June 1982.

99

very critical one, we are still mapping out the territory and are not entirely certain of its dimensions. The problem may be likened to a giant jigsaw puzzle where some of the pieces are missing from the box. Some of the pieces of the puzzle are demographic and others are clinically derived. Sometimes we read about these patients in, or infer their presence from, newspaper accounts (Basler, 1981; Bird, 1981a, 1981b; Herman, 1981). Sometimes there are passing allusions in the professional literature, although very few articles have been devoted exclusively to that population (Bachrach, 1982). Increasingly, now, we seem to hear more and more about young adult chronic patients at national meetings and conferences or wherever mental health professionals convene.

From our pieced-together and still incomplete picture we are beginning to have a sense that the population of young adult chronic mental patients is distributed geographically throughout the nation and is found alike in urban, suburban, and rural communities. From verbal reports, from the scant periodical literature, and from a limited number of official documents and unpublished reports, we know that when these patients are enrolled in psychiatric services they are pervasive users of the service system; they tend to utilize the whole range of psychiatric facilities (Bachrach, 1982). Thus, they are found in state mental hospitals, in community mental health centers, in private psychiatric hospitals, in general hospitals, and in all kinds of outpatient facilities (Bassuk, 1980; Bassuk and Gerson, 1981; Herman, 1981; Kirshner and Ryglewicz, 1980; Lehmann, 1979; Pepper and Ryglewicz, 1980; Platman and Booker, 1981; Robbins and others, 1978; Sheets, 1980). However, at any given time a substantial portion of the target population is not enrolled in psychiatric facilities and is essentially unserved by the psychiatric service system. Growing numbers of young adult chronic mental patients (or would-be patients) are street people (Bird, 1981a, 1981b; New York State Department of Social Services, 1980; Segal and Baumohl, 1980; Segal, Baumohl, and Johnson, 1977).

Those young adult chronic patients utilize the psychiatric service system in a revolving-door manner and move from one facility to another. They frequently become involved in the criminal justice system as well as the psychiatric service system (Basler, 1981). Robbins and his associates (1978) provide a typical description of the population of young adult chronic patients as being in "a state of disequilibrium because they cannot adapt to the community and cannot remain in the hospital. . . . Although their symptoms respond well to the hospital environment, they refuse to remain more than a short time, either requesting discharge or eloping. When in the community they do not participate for long, if at all, in therapeutic programs" (p. 44).

In many communities these patients become general hospital emergency room regulars. Their referral out of the emergency room to other facilities tends to be exceedingly problematic because these patients are difficult to engage in treatment and appear to have no established niche in the psychiatric service system.

In short, young adult chronic mental patients appear to be ubiquitous and very troublesome. They are properly described as chronic patients in that they conform to at least three important criteria of chronicity as described by Peele and Palmer (1980): they have substantial deficits in functioning, they exhibit continued dependency in their life styles, and they show evidence of indefinite need for psychiatric and social support services.

These patients are frequently, but not exclusively, male (Pepper and Ryglewicz, 1980; Robbins and others, 1978); they are frequently, but not exclusively, diagnosed with schizophrenic disorders, although diagnoses of personality disorders appear to be almost as prevalent in some communities (Lehmann, 1979; Pepper and Ryglewicz, 1980; Robbins and others, 1978; Sheets, 1980). Substance abuse is often a contributing factor in their clinical course (Pepper and Ryglewicz, 1980; Robbins and others, 1978).

Few facilities appear to know quite what to do with these young adult patients. Harris and Bergman (1979) from St. Elizabeth's Hospital in Washington write: "After several rounds of bouncing between hospital and community, no one expects these patients to change. They are treated perfunctorily . . . by a staff that is too discouraged to do more than go through the motions" (p. 4). An article by Robbins and others (1978) describes these patients in New York City as surly individuals whom staff perceive as "negativistic, difficult, and frightening" (p. 45).

These descriptions come from metropolitan inner city service settings. But Robert DeForge (personal communication, 1981), the director of Alternate Care Services in Washington County, Vermont, provides a strikingly similar description from a rural portion of the nation. In that community, the young adult chronic patient population consists primarily of transient in-migrants, although some native-born individuals are also included. DeForge indicates that these patients are seen by many service providers as individuals who "will confound all your treatment efforts, who will take your emergency workers and your other treatment people and run them in circles so that the staff reaction to them is basically a lot of anger and frustration."

There is little question that these young adult chronic patients tend to fall squarely within the category of patients described by Chrzanowski (1980) as "problem patients," who are socially unresponsive, hostile, and acting-out individuals with a "high degree of therapeutic immunity." Their complicated patterns of social interaction tend to be affect-laden, so that in therapeutic relationships, they are often characterized by what Chrzanowski (1980) calls "instantaneous transference." In turn, they tend to generate serious counter-transference reactions in their therapists (DeForge, personal communication, 1981).

The increasing prominence of young adult chronic patients results from a variety of factors. In part, they represent the group of individuals who would have been institutionalized twenty-five or thirty years ago. Once admitted to institutions, they would probably have stayed there for the rest of their lives.

They would have become part of a state hospital-based population pool that was essentially static except for new admissions or deaths. Today, however, these individuals, because of deinstitutionalization policies and practices, assume increasing visibility in the psychiatruc service system; they are no longer confined to institutions for life. A sizable number never even enter institutions (New York State Department of Social Services, 1980; Pepper and Ryglewicz, 1980). Others may enter institutions but tend to stay only a short while before they are returned to the community.

However, these young patients are not entirely an artifact of deinstitutionalization. Their increasing numbers in the community are also related to changing demographic conditions in the nation as a whole (Beck and others, 1981). Since these patients are young, and since their disabilities tend to persist, there has been an accumulation of such individuals from successive birth cohorts. This accumulation has been especially marked in recent years, as the postwar baby-boom babies have been reaching maturity. Today the bumper crop of sixty-four million babies who were born between 1946 and 1961 is between the ages of twenty and thirty-five. They represent nearly a third of the nation's population. Because of this overrepresentation, the absolute number of persons at risk for developing schizophrenic or other chronic mental disorders is very substantial. It is no wonder that they constitute such a drain on the psychiatric service system.

What have these young adult chronically mentally ill persons to do with model programs for chronic mental patients? Before proceeding, I should like to clarify the meaning of "model program." *Model* is a word that is used in a number of ways. It may refer to a treatment approach or intervention—for example, a rehabilitation model or a medical model. It may be used as a synonym for the words *good* or *successful* to describe a demonstrably effective program. It may be used to refer to an abstraction or an ideal type—a paradigm, as in a mathematical model. It may be used to describe demonstration or experimental programs. The word *model* is used here exclusively in the latter sense. For purposes of this chapter, a model program is a demonstration effort that tests the application of distinctive, often innovative, program strategies for the care of chronic mental patients.

Model programs are generally, although not necessarily, small in size. Since they are essentially experimental efforts, participants in them are generally selected in accord with the programs' experimental aims. Often funding for these programs is provided by external agencies for the express purpose of testing new procedures or treatments. Although model programs may be found in both institutional and noninstitutional settings, they are most often identified with community-based care. Accordingly, this chapter refers to those that are community-based. Among the better-known model programs for chronic mental patients throughout the country are Fountain House in New York City; Training for Community Living in Madison, Wisconsin; Places for People in St. Louis, Missouri; and Hill House in Cleveland, Ohio.

We must exercise caution in looking to model programs for guidance; we cannot solve the problems of mental health systems in the 1980s by cloning model programs. Although many excellent model programs have been developed for the care of chronic mental patients, they tend to be too focused in their designs and too selective in their service populations to serve as systems solutions. In the simplest terms, the global needs of the mentally ill must be dealt with on a systems level, a level at which model programs do not operate. There are too many chronically ill individuals with too wide a range of disabilities and treatment needs to be served fully by the relatively small number of isolated model programs (Bachrach, 1980b).

Despite this limitation, however, we have learned a great deal from those model programs that have been tested. Those that effectively serve their target populations of chronic mental patients share a number of structural principles that appear to hold, irrespective of the specific locus of care or treatment philosophy, and independently of whether the program is publicly or privately funded (Bachrach, 1980b). There are eight such principles, and together they form a least common denominator of effective program design for chronic mental patients. These eight principles are uniformly present in model programs that are reported to be working successfully for chronic mental patients.

A first principle is that the program assigns top priority to the care of the most severely impaired patients and is targeted toward those who are most persistently ill. If this seems too elementary a principle to merit specific mention, I would only like to point out that the very failure to assign first priority to the most seriously disabled in many community mental health programs has caused major problems for the chronically mentally ill. Chronic mental patients are generally impotent when it comes to advocating on their own behalf, and when they have had to compete for scarce resources with other, less severely impaired patients, they have not tended to fare well.

A second principle is that the program is realistically linked to other resources in the community. This is an affirmation of the range and diversity of treatment needs of chronic mental patients. In a fragmented service system, linkages between the core program and other agencies that serve the patient must be firmly established.

A third principle is that the program, either by itself or in combination with the other resources to which it is linked, attempts to provide for its patients the full range of functions that are associated with institutional care. It acknowledges that chronic mental patients constitute a dependent population for whom the fulfillment of certain basic conditions of human existence must be arranged, conditions that have traditionally, for better or worse, been met within large institutions. To this end, the program is responsive not only to the psychiatric and medical treatment needs of patients but also to their needs for asylum, respite, socialization, and rehabilitation services.

A fourth principle is that the program is tailored to the needs of individual patients. There are personally designed treatment regimens, whether they consist of chemotherapy, psychotherapy, psychosocial rehabilitation, or some combination of these or other treatment modalities. Individual treatment in fact is the cornerstone of effective model programs for chronic mental patients. The principle of reaching out to patients on an individualized basis automatically activates other elements of treatment that are widely understood as fundamental to the care of the chronically mentally ill. Program elements like twenty-four-hour crisis intervention and case management are automatically assumed and assured when the principle of individualized programming is at work. In fact, individualized treatment renders a given program the conceptual opposite of "dumping"—that is, indiscriminate and wholesale placement of patients, either in hospitals or in the community, without consideration for their specific needs.

A fifth principle is that, just as the program is tailored to meet the needs of the individuals it serves, so is it tailored to conform to the local realities of the community in which it is found. It is essential that a program for the chronically mentally ill be compatible with its culture base. Any program may be studied and possibly adapted to some extent to another community's needs, but, basically, every good program for chronic mental patients is local and idiosyncratic.

A sixth principle is that the program emphasizes the need for staff who are attuned to the special survival problems of chronic mental patients living in noninstitutional settings. This principle is of central importance. It has been noted that any program lacking staff "who are trained and comfortable working with disturbed patients in community settings . . . is likely to have poorer outcomes than psychiatric hospitalization" (Polak and Kirby, 1976, p. 21).

A seventh principle is that the program is tied in some manner to a complement of hospital beds. This principle is consistent with the growing view that there are certain patients for whom periods of hospital care continue to be a necessity. Irrespective of what reasons may be considered as appropriate ones for hospitalization—whether for the protection of the patient or society or to provide the patient with diagnostic or intensive treatment service—model programs reflect the ever increasing departure from the polarized antihospital stance that characterized the early years of the deinstitutionalization movement.

An eighth and final principle is that the program has built into it an ongoing internal assessment mechanism that permits ready modifications. This kind of continuous self-monitoring may be and usually is something quite different from formal program evaluation. Computer-assisted program evaluation tends to be too complex, with too slow a turnaround time to be of use in the kind of equilibrating function that is implicit in this principle.

Together these principles are basic to programs that minister to chronic mental patients by acknowledging that they have severe and recurrent problems, that they are frequently functionally impaired and in need of assistance in gaining access to the most basic of life's entitlements, and, most of all, that their individuality is of greater significance in effective treatment than is any categorical label, such as "schizophrenic," that might be applied to them.

Even though model programs are not readily reproducible (they tend to be too culture-bound and too idiosyncratic to be easily reproduced), the eight principles that underlie them have a great deal of generalizability (Bachrach, 1980b). Indeed, these eight principles may be applied to the design of other, even nonmodel, programs for the chronically mentally ill. They are particularly relevant to program planning for the young adult chronically mentally ill target population. They provide a structural framework of necessary, if not sufficient, conditions which must be met if this population is to be served in a sensitive and effective manner. Certain of these principles, in fact, take on particular meaning when they are applied to this special population. The principle of cultural relevance in program planning provides a case in point. Since young adult chronic patients are frequently individuals who are described in a New York State Office of Mental Health (1980) report as "disaffiliated street people," programs for their care should be planned with an appreciation of the uniqueness of street culture, which tends to differ materially from the cultural exposures of most mental health workers. Some of the nuances of street culture include special survival skills, special language, and unique sources of prestige (Bird, 1981a.) Accordingly, Segal and Baumohl (1980) write that, in order to engage California's young patient population in treatment, lengthy paperwork procedures and formal treatment settings should be studiously avoided. And these authors assert that coffeehouses and community "living rooms" work most effectively as treatment settings, because they are "typically open to anyone and are unencumbered by intake and assessment protocols that ritually confirm clienthood and are perceived [by young patients] as threats or create formality and social distance" (p. 363).

The necessity for providing a complement of hospital beds, another of the structural principles identified in model programs for chronic mental patients, also takes on special significance for these young adult patients. Several authorities have noted that, for a variety of reasons, state hospital programs frequently do not meet the needs of these young patients in an era of deinstitutionalization. Young adult patients often fail to utilize state hospitals optimally; they do not tend to benefit greatly from the hospital experience, and tend to leave the hospital against medical advice before they can reap maximum benefits from its services. To the extent that the admission of these patients to state hospitals is not always a desirable alternative, we should be making an effort to utilize hospitals only when they represent the most therapeutic environment (Bachrach, 1980a). It follows that entitlements and benefits for these patients should not be tied in any way to their having undergone a period of care inside a state hospital.

Segal and Baumohl (1980) in California, as well as other writers, stress the importance for young chronic patients of others of these eight principles, such as the need to provide a full range of patient services in community settings and the need to link fragmented resources (Bachrach, 1982). In line with these observations, a *New York Times* article describes a residential facility serving street people, including some young chronic patients, in lower Manhattan (Bird, 1981b). That facility is operated by Franciscan friars, and it provides residents' room and board. It further arranges for the delivery of social, recreational, prevocational, psychiatric, and medical services, including semiweekly visits from physicians at Bellevue Hospital.

But programs like this one are rare. For the most part, young adult chronic mental patients have great difficulty in fitting into established program settings. We have some very special systems problems with these particular patients because they are quintessentially patients who are difficult to treat — apt to be rejected wherever they are found.

In short, mental health systems are not generally designed to treat young adult chronic patients optimally. Segal and Baumohl (1980) refer to these individuals as career mental patients who are destined to become "the most difficult mental patients of the 1980s." They will probably continue to drift within and through the service system and to impose great stresses on it unless a high priority is placed on developing programs for their care.

It seems that, unless special effort is made to integrate the needs of these patients into the system of care, as it has been in Rockland County, New York, these patients will probably be overlooked and rejected (Kirshner and Ryglewicz, 1980; Pepper and Ryglewicz, 1980). Even in Rockland County there are important externally imposed systems constraints; much of the target population is not eligible for certain state Community Support System (CSS) services, such as case management, because they have never had a hospital stay or have had insufficiently long hospital stays. Thus, the system seems, ironically, to reward institutionalism.

It has for some time been our custom to support the development of model programs for chronic mental patients that we then hope to duplicate in a multitude of settings. I believe that it is exceedingly difficult — perhaps even dangerous — to try to transplant entire model programs to alternate settings for several compelling reasons.

For one thing, any program, model or otherwise, has a cultural context. The separation of a program from its culture base can potentially lead to irrelevant or inappropriate programming.

No less important is the fact that many model programs have proceeded with special start-up funds and personnel. Attempts to adapt these programs to the realities of local budgets and resources will inevitably mean cutting out portions of the plan. But we cannot readily foresee the effects of such cuts. Test and Stein (1978), in describing their well-known model program in Madison, Wisconsin, suggest that their own program differs from traditional programs along so many dimensions that it is difficult to sort out "which of the factors carry the greater part of the variance in accounting for the favorable results" (p. 73).

Furthermore, we do not know how much of a specific program's success comes from its having been singled out as a model to be funded and implemented, and how much comes from the actual program elements. Almost certainly, there is a "Hawthorne effect" present in many model programs — a situation in which it is difficult to distinguish the positive effects of the planned program from those that are brought about by the mere fact of being part of an experiment (Bachrach, 1980b).

Another limitation on the reproducibility of model programs comes from the personnel involved. Since model programs tend to attract dedicated and devoted individuals to work in them, positive program results are as likely to come from the ministrations of staff as from the program itself. Precisely who delivers services and the manner in which those services are delivered are of critical importance in the success of any program.

To summarize, it seems to be well nigh impossible to transplant a model program in its entirety to a new setting. And when we try to transplant only portions of programs, it is difficult to know how to select the right program elements for transfer, if, indeed, elements can in fact be separated from their original context with any degree of success.

The limited generalizability of model programs was noted by Suchman (1967), who wrote that every model program is, in effect, the statement of a hypothesis with "almost no generalizability." This is not, of course, an indictment of model programs, but it does suggest that their value lies not in their reproducibility per se, but rather in their scientific yield (Bachrach, 1980b).

Accordingly, it seems to me that the time has come for us to change our perspective. We have devoted so much effort to seeking and developing model programs that we have lost sight of the forest for our preoccupation with the trees. Although we now have considerable knowledge about program principles, we have difficulty in putting that knowledge to work, because we fail to ask big questions, on a systems level. Instead, we persevere with little questions and keep looking for new and better models, while the eight principles of successful programming that we already understand are, in general, ignored in mental health systems planning.

The principles of program planning described here are thrown into bold relief in successful model programs, and this is the basic value of these programs. Because these programs tend to be small and focused in their purposes, and because they are frequently reported in the literature, these principles have become identified with them. But this does not mean that implementation of these principles should be limited to model programs. In fact, the absence of these principles of effective programming from mental health systems is glaringly evident, and we must find ways to incorporate them into systems planning.

We shall not be able to provide for the global treatment needs of young adult chronic mental patients (or, for that matter, any other chronic patients) until we are able to effect some fundamental changes in our program planning practices. We must shift away from the habit of looking to models as solutions and instead move toward integrating some of what is already known into the service delivery practices of mental health systems. This is the challenging task that confronts us as we begin to plan effective programs for the very vulnerable target population of young adult chronic patients.

References

Anonymous. "Cancro Focuses on Functioning of Schizophrenic Youths." *Psychiatric News,* 1981, *5,*

Bachrach, L. L. "Is the Least Restrictive Environment Always the Best?" *Hospital and Community Psychiatry,* 1980a, *31,* 97–102.

Bachrach, L. L. "Overview: Model Programs for Chronic Mental Patients." *American Journal of Psychiatry,* 1980b, *137,* 1023–1031.

Bachrach, L. L. "Young Adult Chronic Patients: An Analytical Review of the Literature." *Hospital and Community Psychiatry,* 1982, *33,* 189–197.

Basler, B. "Assault on Officer and a Drifter's Lack of Treatment." *New York Times,* May 12, 1981.

Bassuk, E. L. "The Impact of Deinstitutionalization on the General Hospital Psychiatric Ward." *Hospital and Community Psychiatry,* 1980, *31,* 623–627.

Bassuk, E. L., and Gerson, S. "Chronic Crisis Patients: A Discrete Clinical Group." *American Journal of Psychiatry,* 1980, *137,* 1513–1517.

Beck, M., Witherspoon, D., Foote, D., Brott, D., Buckley, J., Rogal, K., and Contreras, J. "The Baby Boomers Come of Age." *Newsweek,* March 30, 1981, 34–37.

Bird, D. "Help Is Urged for 36,000 Homeless in City's Streets." *New York Times,* March 8, 1981a.

Bird, D. "Wanderers Find Shelter and a New Life." *New York Times,* April 21, 1981b.

Chrzanowski, G. "Problem Patients or Troublemakers? Dynamic and Therapeutic Considerations." *American Journal of Psychotherapy,* 1980, *34,* 26–34.

Harris, M., and Bergman, H. "Coordination of Inpatient Hospitalization and Community Support Programs: An Integrated Systems Approach." Working paper, St. Elizabeth's Hospital, Washington, 1979 (photocopied).

Herman, R. "Funds Asked for Sites to Contain Violent Patients." *New York Times,* March 8, 1981.

Kirshner, M. C., and Ryglewicz, H. "The Young Adult Chronic Patient: The Rockland County Experience: Case Studies." Presented at the Conference on the Young Adult Chronic Patient, Suffern, N.Y., November, 1980.

Lehmann, J. B. "Mental Health Follow-Up Care Updated." Unpublished manuscript, Elgin Mental Health Center, Elgin, Ill., 1979 (photocopied).

New York State Department of Social Services. "Survey of the Needs and Problems of Single Room Occupancy (SRO) Hotel Residents on the Upper West Side of Manhattan, New York City: Final Report of the SRO Project." Albany, New York, 1980.

New York State Office of Mental Health, Department of Social Services. "New York State's versus New York City's Record in Mental Health and Social Services." Albany, N.Y., 1980.

Peele, R., and Palmer, R. R. "Patient Rights and Patient Chronicity." *Journal of Psychiatry and the Law,* 1980, 59–71.

Pepper, B., and Ryglewicz, H. "The Young Adult Chronic Patient: Keynote Address:

Overview of the Population and the Issues." Presented at the Conference on the Young Adult Chronic Patient, Suffern, N.Y., November 1980.

Platman, S. R., and Booker, T. C. "The Changing Nature of the State Mental Hospital System." Unpublished manuscript, State of Maryland Department of Health and Mental Hygiene, Baltimore, 1981.

Polak, P. R., and Kirby, M. W. "A Model to Replace Psychiatric Hospitals." *Journal of Nervous and Mental Disease,* 1976, *162* (1), 13–22.

Robbins, E., Stern, M., Robbin, L., and others. "Unwelcome Patients: Where Can They Find Asylum?" *Hospital and Community Psychiatry,* 1978, *24,* 44–46.

Segal, S. P., and Baumohl, J. "Engaging the Disengaged: Proposals on Madness and Vagrancy." *Social Work,* 1980, *25* (5), 358–365.

Segal, S. P., Baumohl, J., and Johnson, E. "Falling Through the Cracks: Mental Disorder and Social Margin in a Young Vagrant Population." *Social Problems,* 1977, *24,* 387–400.

Sheets, J. L. "The Hutchings Psychiatric Center Experience: Current Profiles of the Young Adult Chronic Patient at Hutchings and Lessons to be Learned: Conceptual Framework and Data Packet." Presented at the Conference on the Young Adult Chronic Patient, Suffern, N.Y., November 1980.

Suchman, E. A. *Evaluative Research.* New York: Russell Sage Foundation, 1967.

Test, M. A., and Stein, L. I. "Training in Community Living: Research Design and Results." In L. I. Stein and M. A. Test (Eds.), *Alternatives to Mental Hospital Treatment.* New York: Plenum, 1978.

Leona Bachrach is associate professor of psychiatry (sociology)
at the Maryland Psychiatric Research Center, University of Maryland
School of Medicine Department of Psychiatry, Catonsville, Maryland.
She previously served as staff sociologist for the President's Commission
on Mental Health, where she coordinated the Task Panel on
Deinstitutionalization, Rehabilitation, and Long-Term Care.

*A philosopher's perspective, a spontaneous response to presentations
at a conference on the young adult chronic patient, illuminates issues
of mental health and social policy.*

A Philosopher's View

Samuel Gorovitz

I am a philosopher, not a mental health professional; I come to this subject as
an innocent. Philosophy is an obscure discipline in the judgment of most people, intimidating in the judgment of too many. Because I will concern myself
with a discussion about ethics, I will begin by explaining what I mean when I
talk about ethics.

Questions of ethics are not questions of how to practice a profession
without getting sued. Many of the courses in professional ethics these days
seem to have as their implicit motto "Guard Thy Flank." That is not what the
term means to me, nor does it mean sermonizing, telling people how they
ought to behave. It is quite a different matter. Questions of ethics are questions of justice, of fairness, of human dignity, of respect for persons, of virtue,
of integrity — of what, all things considered, is right to do, not in a practical
sense but in a moral sense. Ethics is also reflection on how one ought to be, or
what sort of character one ought to aspire to have. These are elusive concepts,
very difficult to become clear about. That difficulty underlies some of the frustration that is often involved in ethical reflection. It occurred to me as I lis-
tened to the description of some patients and the apparent intractability of
some of them in the face of therapeutic interventions that there are other disci-
plines as frustrating as ethics sometimes can be. This ought on that account to
be a somewhat sympathetic audience, because part of my thesis is that the very
difficult is not necessarily impossible. I would put both ethics and certain kinds
of psychotherapeutic interventions together in that category.

B. Pepper, H. Ryglewicz (Eds.). *New Directions for Mental Health Services: The Young Adult
Chronic Patient,* no. 14. San Francisco: Jossey-Bass, June 1982.

The second point I want to make about ethics is that it is its own thing. Ethics, as I said, is not practical management of one's relationship with the law or potential litigants, nor is ethics simply the deliverance of moral prescription. It is reflection on the difference between right and wrong, an attempt to understand what characterizes morally justifiable behavior and how to separate it from action that is not morally justifiable. That is not the same as law, sociology, history, economics, or any other discipline. With respect to ethical dilemmas, a standard response is to ask, "What does the law say?" What the law says never settles the question. The law is often inadequate to single out a specific course of action. But beyond that, there is always the separate question, "Given that the law says what is legally required, what, all things considered, ought I to do?" Civil disobedience and legal reform both arise out of that point. If law and morality were the same, it would never make sense to argue that some law ought to be changed because it was unjust or morally deficient.

Similarly, ethics isn't sociological inquiry. It is not inquiry into what is typically done; it is not inquiry into history, as the fiddler on the roof suggests when he invokes tradition as the solution to moral conflict. Nor is ethics economics. Often medicine contemplates questions of life extension and the termination of life-support intervention, asking, "Should the plug be pulled?" The cost effectiveness answer is typically "Yes." It is almost always cheaper. But that kind of crude economic analysis or even a fairly sophisticated economic analysis always falls short of giving us a satisfying answer to the puzzlement about what we ought to do. These remarks simply underscore that ethics is an autonomous discipline.

I have not claimed that questions of law or economics or sociology or psychology or history are ethically irrelevant, only that they are not ethically determinant. So the basic question is "What ought I to do? How ought I to behave?" And that question becomes interesting when it arises in the context of conflict. There are many situations where we have no moral puzzlement. We can often view a type of behavior as perhaps saintly or perhaps morally repugnant without any sense of conflict, either collectively or intrapersonally. For example, puppy punting is easy to agree upon as morally repugnant behavior, like mugging octogenarian pensioners for sport, or boiling babies for bouillon. There is no shortage of clear examples of behavior with respect to which there is no moral conflict. That is not to say that one cannot make a moral judgment about them. It is to say that the moral judgment that one makes about them is simple and uncontroversial. Ethics comes into play where moral conflict occurs.

Why does moral conflict occur? Under what sorts of circumstances? It arises because we cannot have what we want; often the world is recalcitrant. It arises in connection with scarcity of all sorts, and the resultant uncertainty about how we should distribute and allocate the good things. "The good things" do not necessarily mean material things. I mean goods and opportunities of every sort — positions of influence, access to education, the distribution of one's time or one's affections. Anything that is valued — material, social, or interpersonal — is scarce, and hence allocation problems arise. Conflicts are potentially present, and it is the resolution of those conflicts that generates problems of distributive justice. That kind of context gives rise to ethical conflict.

A second kind of conflict has to do with diversity in valuation of goals, of ends to be achieved. Very often two people are in conflict because they are acting in pursuit of different objectives. They might agree entirely about what one ought to do in order to get from where they are to any one of a number of different end points, but what they disagree about is destination. Such conflict with respect to goal valuation is a major source of ethical conflict — conflict of values. Another source of ethical conflict has to do with the perception that the ends, once agreed upon, are achievable only by means that are in some respect distasteful. The question then is of what sorts of compromises one is willing to make between what one wants to achieve and how one wants to act. These conflicts, it is important to emphasize, are not merely interpersonal. We are all very aware of interpersonal conflict of an ethical sort if we think about socially divisive issues such as abortion policy. It is common that we have a sea of partisans each of whom has a confident apprehension of the true moral view and views everyone else as morally pathological. (Of course, there are some people who find dissenters from their view to be not merely different, but morally repugnant.)

There is, therefore, a social policy problem: How do we make a collective decision in a context of pluralism of values? But if that were all ethics had to deal with, it would be a much easier discipline than it is. The problems run deeper, because the very same conflicts that we see mirrored in social diversity are conflicts that can be intrapersonal. People are often ambivalent about ethically divisive cases, and they see and identify with incompatible points of view simultaneously. So the same kind of conflict that gives rise to philosophical reflection about the distinction between right and wrong also can be anxiety producing. It has its psychological dimension. Ethics is in part a response to moral anxiety.

I want to say a bit about the subject matter of ethics, and then try to link some of those notions with the issues that have been raised here. There are essentially two basic moral traditions that have flourished over the last two thousand years — which is not really long when you consider the history of human activity. (I point that out because some people get impatient with the fact that the philosophers have not got all the answers fashioned yet.) Those two moral traditions, which are the most significant, the most persistent, and the most dominant, are the consequentialist tradition and the nonconsequentialist tradition. I hope you will appreciate the completeness of that way of partitioning the world.

The consequentialist tradition is represented most famously by John Stuart Mill, in the little pamphlet *Utilitarianism,* originally a series of four magazine articles. Mill's view is that the right thing to do is that which produces the greatest good for the greatest number. It is as simple as that. The simplicity is illusory; it turns out to be excruciatingly complicated to make sense of that moral position. But on the face of it, anyway, it is relatively clear. It says that morality is future-oriented, that it is action-oriented, that it is consequence-oriented; that the right thing to do is the thing which will yield the right kind of payoff, where the payoff is defined in terms of what is very much the psychiatrists' stock in trade—human happiness and the balance of happiness over suffering.

But that is not the only moral theory that is prominent. The nonconsequentialist theories are exemplified by, for example, the Ten Commandments. The Ten Commandments, or any other list of commandments you like, are not future-oriented; they are not consequentialist. They say, "Here are some categories of behavior that are forbidden, and here are some categories which are required." One does not ask, "What will happen if I do this?" Instead one asks, "What kind of thing is this to do?" That is a very different view of morality. That view does not have to be rooted in theological traditions, or linked to the Ten Commandments. In fact, there are many different varieties of nonconsequentialist view. The most significant in the history of moral philosophy is probably that advocated by Immanuel Kant. A part of his view can be captured very simply. He says obligations are categorical. If you have made a promise, you must keep it because it is a promise, and that is an end to that. There is no question in the Kantian moral view of calculating what in this instance the result will be of keeping or breaking this particular promise. One can imagine a utilitarian saying, "Yes, I know I promised, and I know that in general it is good to keep one's promises, but in this case lots of harm will be done if I don't break my promise and lots of good will result if I do, so the consequences will be best if I break my promise." That is a completely different kind of approach to the distinction between right and wrong.

Kant said that the fundamental undergirding of all morality is that human beings are ends unto themselves, each separately possessed of human dignity, none ever justifiably used solely as a means toward the objective of someone else. Kant is misquoted as saying, "Never use people as means." He knew better. What Kant said is never to use people as means only, but always to recognize them as autonomous ends unto themselves.

I suggest, and I will try to explain why this is the case, that a lot of your sense of conflict about what to do results from the fact that you think Mill is right, and you think Kant is right, and you think they are incompatible, and you do not know how to get out of that bind.

Some people have criticized moral philosophy, saying, "Isn't it about time you folks settled which one was correct or, failing that, invented some new way of adjudicating the tension between the two or some entirely new and better approach to reflection about moral conflict?" The problem is that the moral relevance of consequentialist considerations cannot justifiably be denied. What happens is morally relevant. But it is similarly undeniable that we nearly all are convinced that consequences alone do not settle the issue. There are some kinds of behavior which are so repugnant morally, and others which are so required morally, that there is a heavy burden of proof that falls to anyone who wants to deviate from those prescriptions — and that burden of proof cannot be borne simply by a facile invocation of the consequences. It is not just that you think Mill is right when you are thinking about Mill, and you think Kant is right when you are thinking about Kant. There really is much merit in each of these views, despite the incompatibility. The mistake is to think that because they are incompatible, one of them has to be wrong.

I want to begin to apply these considerations very gently to mental health interventions. What are some of the issues that would be interesting to pursue seriously if we had any significant time to do it? What goals should you be pursuing? What are the valuable end states toward which your efforts should be directed? I do not think the answer is obvious. You must ask, what are the barriers to the achievement of those goals, and in particular, what are the morally interesting barriers? And finally, what justifies your doing what you do?

I should like to begin with the question of what goals to pursue. A lot of the discussion here seems to be infused with the notion that the patient's best interest motivates what you do. I think it is dishonest to pretend that is the sole goal or the sole motivation. It is wrong also to argue that it ought to be the sole goal. It is important instead to look honestly and clearly at what the various goals and motivations are that interplay. Sometimes what you do is done explicitly in order to help the patient. But sometimes it is to alleviate what are symptoms only because they are not accepted. They are behaviors which are not accepted in the context from which the patient comes, and the intervention then is directed at alleviating the discomfort that others have in dealing with the behavior of the patient. The difference between illness and eccentricity is a question of what the traffic will bear, and sometimes the interventions are motivated not so much solely to benefit the individual, but because the larger context has had enough. I do not think that is an illegitimate motivation. What is illegitimate is to pretend that it is being done solely for the benefit of the patient. There is another dimension of confusion here. People who have sophisticated skills — highly talented, well-trained people — love to do their thing. This is perhaps most obvious in a context like neonatal intensive care. Think about chess and checkers. People who know both games are not likely to be playing checkers. People like to use their most highly developed skills and to meet challenges. I suggest that a lot of the motivation for interventions in medicine is the aesthetic satisfaction of doing the thing — of using the skill, of facing and meeting the challenge. I do not know to what extent that is operative in mental health interventions, but it is a question that it is dishonest to avoid.

There is a tension explicitly mentioned by Stein (see Chapter Seven, this volume) about the relative distribution of benefits and burdens resulting from deinstitutionalization and new modes of interacting with patients of various types. He suggested that it might be future generations of patients who would be the beneficiaries of decisions made about those who are patients today. One of the conflicts that is socially most interesting and important in making a policy decision concerns how we manage the distribution of benefits and of burdens. A lot of what we do in social decision making involves trying to get some measure of the benefits of an action and some measure of the costs (it is even called cost-benefit analysis) and compare them. But that is a very superficial approach. It may well be that the benefits exceed the costs, but that the benefits go to one class of people and the costs are imposed on another class of people. And, therefore, the magnitude of the benefits does not by itself justify the imposition of the costs. So you always have to ask, when you are in the cost-benefit mode, not just what the magnitudes are, but also what the distributions are. A separate question then arises that is very intriguing. To what extent is it justifiable to sacrifice the interests of people with whom we are presently interacting in the interest of a better state for other people elsewhere or subsequently? For the utilitarian, the consequentialist, the answer is straightforward. You are interested only in magnitudes; you are interested only in maximizing payoff. But for the nonconsequentialist, that analysis will not work. And for those of us who embody a mix of both of these tendencies — probably nearly all of us — the problem is particularly acute.

But assume for the moment that your motivation is focused solely on the interest of the patient, that it is unsullied by concern with social benefits apart from the benefit to the individual. What objectives is it reasonable for you to pursue? The World Health Organization tells us that health is not merely the absence of illness or injury, but a complete state of physical, psychological, and social well-being — a spectacular agenda for health care providers. Quite apart from the question of whether you have the requisite expertise to see to it that every dimension of one's life is flourishing, it conjures up all sorts of images, such as the lonely patient for whom you prescribe a computer dating service. Why stop at dating skills? Why not actually provide the dates? Send them to a disco; send Blue Cross the bill! That sounds as though I have said it in jest, but there is a very serious issue here that has been raised repeatedly in the last two days of the conference. That is, how much are you after? What is it that you are aiming to bring about? We all know that there are limitations in the practice of the art. But I am talking now not about what you can actually do, but what you ought to be aiming for. Is it the objective of mental health interventions to make people happy? What are the justifiable goals? I do not think we can begin to wrestle with the question of what the appropriate means are until we are clear about what the goals are toward which we are directing the means.

At this point, I want to turn to the quiet-desperation issue, about which far too much has been said. At least three speakers at the conference said that the mass of men lead lives of quiet desperation. I find that a tendentious description of the state of mankind. Most people at some time or other, and perhaps much of the time, know quiet desperation. That is a fact. But to cite it as a characterization of the human experience seems to me to have unfortunate consequences for mental health goal selection.

The mass of men lead lives of intermittent elation. And there is much more that can be said about the lives that people lead. To say, as if characterizing those lives, that Thoreau got it right seems to me to adopt a rather gloomy approach to human existence that I do not share and that I would lament to see embraced within the mental health professions or any other segment of society. If quiet desperation is viewed as the norm toward which you hope to enable your patients to approach, in contrast with the howling desperation with which they come to you, you are going to have a very limited sense of an appropriate outcome.

Now let me reveal my own prejudice in this matter. I think the mental health profession's proper goal is maximizing functional autonomy in your patients, making it as possible as it can be for them to lead the lives they choose to lead—whether those be lives of stability or lives of wide swings of mood, including the extremes of howling desperation and intermittent elation. I would be loath to endorse the presumption that a stable life of quiet desperation is a better outcome for everyone than a life of instability including a lot of pain and a lot of achievement. To make this more explicit, the appropriate goal is dependent upon the particular individual and what kinds of aspirations that individual has. Since they are all ends unto themselves and ought to be constantly viewed as such, we cannot know, unless we know the individuals and who they are, what is an acceptable outcome or goal for them.

What are the barriers to the achievement of such goals? First, the limitations of the art—the limitations in the knowledge of what the processes are that give rise to disability of the sorts that have been focused on at the conference. But that is not the only barrier. Another is the moral constraint you feel when you believe you can do some good for someone, but only by manipulation and perhaps coercion. You are motivated to make things better for the patient, but you recognize that the patient is somebody after all—someone with rights, with autonomy, with dignity. You first try to suggest, then to persuade, then perhaps to urge most vehemently. Perhaps you go the final step and commit the patient, take over totally the patient's ability to make decisions about the management of his own affairs. But as the level of intervention increases, so, I submit, for most of us does discomfort at overriding that individual's autonomy, and we recognize that only very special justifications allow us to act even in the interest of someone else when in doing so we obliterate their autonomy. Such action is called paternalistic action. (It ought more properly to be called parentalistic.)

If you have a four-year-old child who is running after a ball into the path of an oncoming truck, you don't say, "Child, give me please the opportunity to engage in rational discourse with you — a kind of constructive alliance — about the behavioral decisions you are making. Let me persuade you autonomously and of your own free will to modify your behavior." You grab the kid, yank him out of the street, obliterate his autonomy. Not only is it justifiable, you are morally culpable if you do not do it. So paternalism is not only sometimes justifiable, it is sometimes obligatory. The difficulty is particularly acute when the population that you are talking about is both adult and childlike — at least in certain ways. They have rights, and we recognize that people have the right to act as they see fit not merely when their choices correspond to our preferences and our wise judgment, but otherwise as well.

Freedom is hollow indeed if it is nothing more than freedom to act in a way that will be approved of by others. If we respect the freedom of individuals, we must respect their right to commit folly or to flourish. So we let people do all sorts of loony things, such as hang-gliding or smoking — well, that's a special case because that is not only self-destructive, but often antisocial in a way that hang-gliding is not. But people can be test pilots, can ski down sheer precipices, and can do all sorts of things that we are quite confident are going to get them into trouble. We let people marry others who we know will be bad for them. We try to persuade them; we fail; we stand back. We don't send each of them phony letters of abuse over the other's signature.

There are serious limits on the justifiability of paternalistic intervention. It is important to understand that it is not enough that you be right. All sorts of special conditions have to be satisfied. Otherwise, you have simply violated the autonomy of another human being, and that is morally unjustifiable. Depending upon the particular pattern of violation, it may be legally culpable as well. So the question that rises to the surface is: To what extent are we justified in overriding the autonomy of someone because of our belief that doing so will benefit that person? The conflict we feel results from our desire to provide the benefit and our aversion to violating the autonomy. There is no hope of finding a solution that is permanently comfortable, because whatever decision we make, we make it at some moral cost. When you intervene and override someone's autonomy — give him medication against his will in order to improve his circumstances, for example — you do so with regret at the moral price you had to pay to achieve those good consequences. Or, if you respect the autonomy and let him wallow in his own disability, you respect that autonomy at a price, and you regret the price you have had to pay in lost benefit. The conflict is between our instinct to do good and our instinct to do right; they are different matters.

At this point it may be instructive to remember what Mill had to say about paternalistic intervention. Mill thought there was in general no justification for imposing on anyone else your judgment about what is best for him. But there was one important exception. Mill believed that the ability to act independently in one's own behalf was extremely important. He did believe that it was justifiable to intervene in someone else's affairs, restricting that person's autonomy — as we do with the child whom we grab from the street — but only when what is at issue is the enhancement or preservation of that individual's future autonomy. That is, the sole justification for limiting autonomy is autonomy itself. So you may not intervene in someone else's affairs, according to this analysis, simply because you think the person will be socially more congenial, or even happier, but only because you see the intervention as increasing that individual's future ability to function autonomously. This is to say that one may limit freedom only in the interest of a greater subsequent freedom.

Let me talk briefly about freedom. You hear a lot about freedom, an important concept that divides straightforwardly into two separate notions. We talk about freedom to do this and to do that. We are free to speak our minds; we are free to travel about from place to place; we are free to leave. When we say "It's a free country," what we mean presumably is that we enjoy a variety of freedoms to act in various ways — liberties. The other side of the coin is freedom from — freedom from barriers; freedom from deprivation; freedom from constraints. If an individual's freedom is important because autonomy requires having the ability to be captain of his own destiny, then I suggest that being free to express one's views, travel about, and make one's own decisions, although important, is no more important than being free from the disabilities that result from extreme poverty, extreme illness, extreme hunger, or perhaps extreme psychiatric constraints.

What policies might one want to adopt in the attempt to resolve some of these tensions? It is difficult to know what to say. It does strike me as bizarre that we think involuntary commitment is justifiable when we do not think milder measures are justifiable. It is not easy to justify involuntary commitment, but surely there are cases where it is justifiable, in the interest either of protection of people from clear and present danger or in the interest of replacing a very high degree of dysfunction with some prospect of enhanced autonomy. Of course, that is a small subset of the reasons which historically have been involved in involuntary commitment. Why then should it not be justifiable to invoke a much milder measure — involuntary participation in treatment protocols that are less confining than total commitment? That seems to me a puzzle, the answer to which wholly escapes me. I should end with a question; it would be philosophically inappropriate to do otherwise: Why is there a distinction between the very severe large-scale deprivation of liberty that the mental health professionals think is justifiable, and the rather moderate intermittent limitation of liberty that for the most part seems not to be viewed as justifiable as a mental health intervention?

Samuel Gorovitz is professor and chairman of the department of philosophy at the University of Maryland and has written Doctors' Dilemmas: Moral Conflict and Medical Care *(Macmillan, 1982).*

Two major initiatives in programming and service delivery are proposed for the attention and advocacy efforts of the mental health professions.

Concluding Comments

Bert Pepper
Hilary Ryglewicz

In these closing pages we will address two major aspects of programming and service delivery for the young adult chronic patient, both requiring initiatives on the part of mental health planners at each level of government, and both requiring active advocacy efforts for patients in the community.

As noted repeatedly throughout this volume, even our state-of-the-art community service networks face major problems in providing for the needs of the young adult chronic patient. In Rockland County, which has a rich mix of integrated programs, we still have young adult patients falling through the cracks, and we still have difficulty maintaining continuity of care. In metropolitan settings presenting overwhelming dimensions of unmet human need, our therapeutic tasks must wait until fundamental problems of shelter and survival are addressed. As professionals and as citizens, we cannot help but see, not only the psychiatric disorders of our functionally disabled young adults, but the hazards and shortcomings of life in the communities where they struggling to survive. Some of our patients, who have experienced extreme difficulties in community living, prefer to remain in mental hospitals indefinitely.

A colleague in a state hospital system said recently that his hospital has accumulated a small but significant number of young adults who persistently refuse to be discharged. He said: "Every time we start talking about a sheltered apartment and a day program, these patients become psychotic. They say, 'Look, I know I'm schizophrenic and nothing can be done for me. What's

B. Pepper, H. Ryglewicz (Eds.). *New Directions for Mental Health Services: The Young Adult Chronic Patient*, no. 14. San Francisco: Jossey-Bass, June 1982.

the use of leaving the hospital again, since I'll never make it outside, and I'll only be brought back here?'"

What can we do to make a livable world outside the hospital for these people? The first initiative we need to take is fiscal and therefore political in its nature. This is the allocation or reallocation of mental hygiene resources to offer support to community run programs on a scale with the numbers and nature of patient populations that have become a community responsibility. Such programs now are responsible, clinically and in terms of other human services, for enormous numbers of young adult and other patients who have been discharged from state institutions across the country. This means that our community programs now treat and support groups of patients who, in both their numbers and the severity of their disorders, place demands on us that far exceed our original mandate and funding. Yet community programs typically have not received the benefit of a commensurate shift in resources to support the care of these patients.

This discrepancy is particularly marked in the case of our young adult patient population, who are not a deinstitutionalized but an uninstitutionalized generation. In New York State, for one example, Community Support Services (CSS) funding has been provided for certain community programs, but only for those patients who are eligible based on three hospitalizations of at least ten days each within the past two years; or three months cumulative hospitalization within the past two years; or six months consecutive hospitalization in a person's lifetime. In our initial study of nearly 300 chronically disabled young adults, we found that 25 percent had never been hospitalized, and a total of 55 percent had not spent sufficient time in psychiatric hospitals to be CSS eligible. These outworn eligibility criteria discriminate against (1) patients who are successful in staying out of the hospital and (2) communities where a service network which is effective in helping them stay out has been developed. These criteria prevent many of these young adults from receiving case management and other services which we see as a crucial support to their functioning in community life.

This is one example in one state of the way in which methods of resource allocation are based on conditions and policies which are no longer relevant. On a larger scale, we must address the inequity that continues to exist in many or most states between the resources devoted to the old institutional system and the resources devoted to the newer community system of care. This does not necessarily mean the wholesale abolition of institutions nor wholesale withdrawal of their funding. What it does mean is that new methods of allocating resources must be worked out in such a way that community programs — and community patients — receive equitable treatment. This reallocation of resources and redesigning of our systems for a new era is a prerequisite to the development of more effective services for the young adult and other seriously disabled patient populations.

The second and equally necessary initiative we must take is for the development of a network of community residences and group homes specifically for young adults. Most of the functions of the mental institutions were not in fact medical, but were family and community functions: the provision of food, shelter, protection, socialization, and recreation. Our psychiatrically disabled young adults are not retained in hospitals today because they do not need a hospital level of medical care, but the other supportive, family and community functions still need to be provided in some form for large numbers of these functionally impaired persons. The needs of our young adult chronic patients typically include: (1) a place to live; (2) a close and continuous relationship to a constant clinical staff member or mini-team; (3) a carefully tailored network of supportive vocational and social treatment programs; and (4) a source of help for themselves and their families as they try to work through the painful issues of separation from the family and of disappointed expectations on both sides.

We believe that, for many, these needs could be met effectively through community residences designed specifically for young adults. The functions involved would not be terribly different from the work of an adolescent group home or residential treatment center. We need to provide some alternative to the beleaguered family, to the proprietary home inhabited by older deinstitutionalized patients, to the single room occupancy, and to the streets. We need to provide programs of total care that would occupy a middle ground between the street and the hospital, where disabled young adults could be helped to survive and to grow into, perhaps a compromised, but at least a stable and tolerable, pattern of social functioning.

Deinstitutionalization and outpatient programs in our new era of community care will stand or fall on our success with this young adult population. At the present time we know more than we do; we have more and better guidelines for treatment and programming than we are currently able to put into practice. Much of what we know is fragmented and needs to be gathered together in the form of comprehensible programs. Much of what we do is fragmented because it does not rest upon a solid and continuous foundation of services offering both treatment and provision for fundamental needs. It would be nice to have our solutions rush to us in the form of new medications, major breakthroughs, panaceas — but we cannot simply await miracles. "In the absence of angels, men and women must take their place."

We must test the efficacy of community care by making use of all we know. We must approach the problem of the young adult chronic patient with multimodality, multicomponent plans which reflect, not a passionate commitment to one answer or one solution, but an eclectic attitude, a mature blending of the therapeutic resources available to us, tailored to the needs of individuals and mindful of the full range of those needs. We must continue to bring the magnitude of the problem to the attention of government, the professional community and the public, and we must not rest our case until adequate support is provided for the young adult chronic patient.

Bert Pepper is a psychiatrist, director of the Rockland County Community Mental Health Center, Pomona, New York, clinical professor of psychiatry at New York University, and chairman of the New York State Conference of Local Mental Hygiene Directors.

Hilary Ryglewicz, ACSW, is clinical assistant to the director at the Rockland County Community Mental Health Center.

Index

A

Advisory Social Service Committee of the Municipal Lodging House, 35, 40
Aiello, J. J., 82, 83
Akinesia, and psychopharmacology, 54
Albany Institute for Education and Training, and conference, 1
Allen, P., 57, 66
Alvin, case of, 38
American Medical Association, 47
American Psychiatric Association, 47
Anderson, C. M., 92, 97
Anderson, N., 33, 40
Anonymous, 108
Autonomy: and breakdown in functioning, 9-10; issues of, 117-118

B

Bachrach, L. L., 2, 26, 29, 30-31, 99-109
Bahr, H. M., 33, 34, 40
Basler, B., 100, 108
Bassuk, E. L., 31, 69, 75, 85, 89, 100, 108
Baumohl, J., 4, 13, 31, 35, 41, 100, 105-106, 109
Baxter, E., 1, 33-42
Beck, M., 102, 108
Beels, C. C., 92, 96-97
Bellak, L., 73, 75
Bellevue Hospital, and patients, 26-27, 106
Bendiner, E., 33, 41
Bene-Kocemba, A., 22
Bennett, C. L., 46n
Benson, E., 20
Bergman, H., 101, 108
Berkeley, California, patients in, 26, 105
Berkowitz, R., 92, 97
Bird, D., 100, 105, 106, 108
Birley, J. L., 97
Booker, T. C., 100, 109
Brandon, S., 13
Bristol, J. H., 27, 29, 31
Bronx Psychiatric Center, 92

Brott, D., 108
Brown, G. W., 92, 97
Buckley, J., 108
Burgess, A. W., 71, 73, 75

C

California, patients in, 26, 27-28, 105
Caplan, G., 70, 75
Caton, C. L. M., 8, 13, 25-31, 35, 41
Chafetz, L., 35, 41
Chlorpromazine, 51
Chronicity, defined, 16
Chrzanowksi, G., 101, 108
Cleveland, Ohio, model program in, 102
Clozapine, 55
Cole, R., 22
Community: assertive approach to, 63; development of residences and group homes in, 123; principles for treatment in, 59-66; principles of working with, 63-66; programs in, 58; resources in, use of, 63-64, 103; support and education to, 64-65; treatment of young adults in, 57-67
Community Mental Health Services Act of 1954 (New York), 44
Connecticut, patients in, 27
Contreras, J., 108
Cost-benefit analysis, and goals, 116
Cotton, P. G., 22
Cox, S., 1, 33-42
Creedmoor State Hospital, 51
Crisis, definition of, 70-71
Crisis intervention: assessment for, 71-73; case example of, 71-72; full time, 62; prerequisites for, outpatient, 73-74; therapeutic alliance in, 72-73; with young adults, 69-75

D

Dane County, Wisconsin, community treatment in, 57-67
Davis, E. B., 29, 31
DeForge, R., 101

125